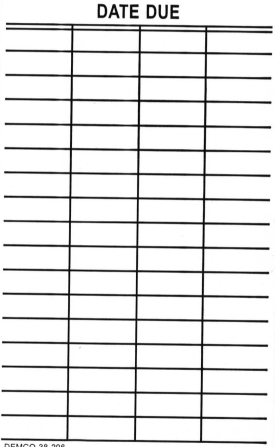

DATE DUE

DEMCO 38-296

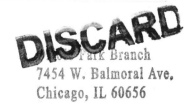

The Skeletal and Muscular System

Titles in the Understanding the Human Body series include:

Understanding
THE HUMAN BODY

The Skeletal and Muscular System

Pam Walker and Elaine Wood

LUCENT
BOOKS ®

THOMSON
———— ✳ ————™
GALE

San Diego • Detroit • New York • San Francisco • Cleveland • New Haven, Conn. • Waterville, Maine • London • Munich

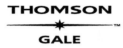

For more information, contact
Lucent Books
27500 Drake Rd.
Farmington Hills, MI 48331-3535
Or you can visit our Internet site at http://www.gale.com

LIBRARY OF CONGRESS CATALOGING-IN-PUBLICATION DATA

Walker, Pam, 1958–
  The skeletal and muscular system / by Pam Walker and Elaine Wood.
    v. cm. — (Understanding the human body)
Includes bibliographical references and index.
Contents: Skeletal system—The muscular system—The joints of the body—Diseases and disorders of the musculoskeletal system—Advances in medical technology on the musculoskeletal front.
  ISBN 1-59018-334-7 (hardback : alk. paper)
1. Musculoskeletal system—Diseases—Juvenile literature. 2. Musculoskeletal system—Juvenile literature. [1. Muscular system. 2. Skeleton.] I. Wood, Elaine, 1950– II. Title. III. Series.
QP301 .W277 2003
612.7—dc21

2002152980

Printed in the United States of America

CONTENTS

FOREWORD

Since Earth first formed, countless creatures have come and gone. Dinosaurs and other types of land and sea animals all fell prey to climatic shifts, food shortages, and myriad other environmental factors. However, one species—human beings—survived throughout tens of thousands of years of evolution, adjusting to changes in climate and moving when food was scarce. The primary reason human beings were able to do this is that they possess a complex and adaptable brain and body.

The human body is comprised of organs, tissue, and bone that work independently and together to sustain life. Although it is both remarkable and unique, the human body shares features with other living organisms: the need to eat, breathe, and eliminate waste; the need to reproduce and eventually die.

Human beings, however, have many characteristics that other living creatures do not. The adaptable brain is responsible for these characteristics. Human beings, for example, have excellent memories; they can recall events that took place twenty, thirty, even fifty years earlier. Human beings also possess a high level of intelligence. Their unique capacity to invent, create, and innovate has led to discoveries and inventions such as vaccines, automobiles, and computers. And the human brain allows people to feel and respond to a variety of emotions. No other creature on Earth has such a broad range of abilities.

Although the human brain physically resembles a large, soft walnut, its capabilities seem limitless. The brain controls the body's movement, enabling humans to sprint, jog, walk, and crawl. It controls the body's internal functions, allowing people to breathe and maintain a heartbeat without effort. And it controls a person's creative talent, giving him or her the ability to write novels, paint masterpieces, or compose music.

Like a computer, the brain runs a network of body systems that keep human beings alive. The nervous system relays the brain's messages to the rest of the body. The respiratory system draws in life-sustaining oxygen and expels carbon dioxide waste. The circulatory system carries that oxygen to and from the body's vital organs. The reproductive system allows humans to continue their species and flourish as the dominant creatures on the planet. The digestive system takes in vital nutrients and converts them into the energy the body needs to grow. And the immune system protects the body from disease and foreign objects. When all of these systems work properly, the result is an intricate, extraordinary living machine.

Even when some of the systems are not working properly, the human body can often adapt. Healthy people have two kidneys, but, if necessary, they can live with just one. Doctors can remove a defective liver, heart, lung, or pancreas and replace it with a working one from another body. And a person blinded by an accident, disease, or birth defect can live a perfectly normal life by developing other senses to make up for the loss of sight.

The human body adapts to countless external factors as well. It sweats to cool off, adjusts the level of oxygen it needs at high altitudes, and derives nutritional value from a wide variety of foods, making do with what is available in a given region.

Only under tremendous duress does the human body cease to function. Extreme fluctuations in temperature, an invasion by hardy germs, or severe physical damage can halt normal bodily functions and cause death. Yet, even in such circumstances, the body continues to try to repair itself. The body of a diabetic, for example, will take in extra liquid and try to expel excess glucose through the urine. And a body exposed to extremely low temperatures will shiver in an effort to generate its own heat.

Lucent's Understanding the Human Body series explores different systems of the human body. Each volume describes the parts of a given body system and how they work both individually and collectively. Unique characteristics, malfunctions, and cutting edge medical procedures and technologies are also discussed. Photographs, diagrams, and glossaries enhance the text, and annotated bibliographies provide readers with opportunities for further discussion and research.

▌ The Skeletal System

Movement is an adaptation that is central to the survival of many organisms. The ability to move makes it possible to relocate to a better habitat, find a new source of food, or get out of the range of a predator. Movement is so significant that living things have developed a variety of ways to accomplish it.

Under the microscope, the amoeba, a one-celled creature, looks similar to a spot of jelly. This tiny organism, or microbe, moves by extending a portion of its body forward. The rest of the cell then flows into the extension, and repeated "extend and flow" cycles pull the microbe along at a slow but reliable rate. Other one-celled microbes have specialized structures that help them move. Cilia, which look like tiny hairs, stick out from cell membranes of microorganisms called paramecia. In most cases, cilia act like tiny oars that paddle organisms through their fluid surroundings. Alternately, however, they create swirls in the liquid environment, sweeping food into the microbe's mouthlike opening. Still other types of microbes use different yet effective means of locomotion.

Animals are larger and more complex than one-celled creatures, so the mechanisms that enable them to move are also more complicated. The bodies of animals are equipped with muscles, specialized tissues that can contract and relax. Muscles are essential for animal movement, but they need help. Muscles must have a rigid structure against which to push. A skeleton meets this requirement.

Skeletal Types

Skeletons come in different shapes and sizes. Many small, simple animals like sea anemones and earthworms have hydrostatic skeletons. *Hydro* refers to fluid and aptly describes a skeleton made of a tubelike structure filled with fluid. Like an inflated balloon, a hydrostatic skeleton is firm and provides a hard surface against which muscles can push. Animals that possess hydrostatic skeletons generally do not move rapidly or with great grace; nevertheless, they successfully get from one place to another.

More complex small animals are covered with close-fitting but rigid exoskeletons. Exoskeletons protect the body like armor and provide excellent support against which muscles can push, thus allowing faster and more precise movements

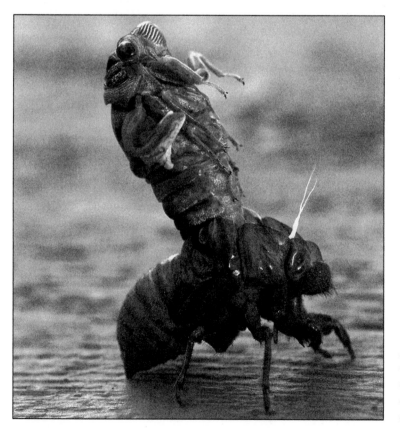

Like other insects, a cicada sheds its exoskeleton to allow for growth of a new, larger one.

than other types of skeletons. The exoskeletons of dragonflies enable them to perform remarkable feats such as hovering, darting, and soaring. Crickets, fleas, and some jumping spiders, all equipped with exoskeletons, are able to propel themselves to great heights, often hundreds of times their own body length.

Despite their great assets, exoskeletons have some disadvantages. As the muscles and other flexible tissues of an organism grow, its stiff, unchanging exoskeleton becomes too small. Therefore, the animal must shed its outgrown suit and produce a new, larger one. During periods of shedding, when the animal is relatively unprotected, it is vulnerable to attack from predators.

The skeletons of humans and other complex animals are made primarily of bone found inside the body. These structures, called endoskeletons, serve as internal frameworks, like the wooden supports that provide the framing of a house. In the animal kingdom, animals with internal skeletons are in the minority, representing less than 5 percent of the animals on Earth.

Skeletons in the Closet and Out

The term *skeleton* comes from the Greek word for "dried up body." Even though animal bones found in the desert are dry and brittle, the bone making up a skeleton in a living organism is alive and dynamic. The outer, compact layer of a living bone is very dense and strong. On the inside, bone is filled with spongy, lightweight material that resembles a honeycomb. The central shaft of some bones contains marrow, a jellylike material.

Bone is not simply a fixture against which muscle can work; it plays several important roles in the body. It is a support system that holds up the body, giving it shape and form. Like the steel girders of a skyscraper, the skeleton of a human holds the other body structures in place. Bone also surrounds and protects internal organs. The bones that form the chest and the back shield the heart, lungs, and other chest organs from damage. The internal cavities of bones provide a place where some fat is stored. Certain bones store fat in their marrow, while others contain material that makes new blood cells. And bone stores vital minerals, especially calcium and magnesium.

A newborn baby has about 350 individual bones, many of which fuse together as they grow. An adult human body contains only 206 different bones, accounting for about 20 percent of the individual's body weight.

Not all bones look alike; they vary greatly in size and structure. A bone is generally classified into one of four basic shapes: long, short, flat, and irregular. The long bones are found in arms and legs, whereas some of the shortest are in the fingers and toes. Most of the bones that make up the skull are flat, and those that support the face are irregular.

Life as a Bone

The long part of a bone is called the shaft, or diaphysis. The outer portion of the shaft is very tight, compact bone that is covered by a tough, protective tissue called the periosteum. The areas at the ends of long bones are the

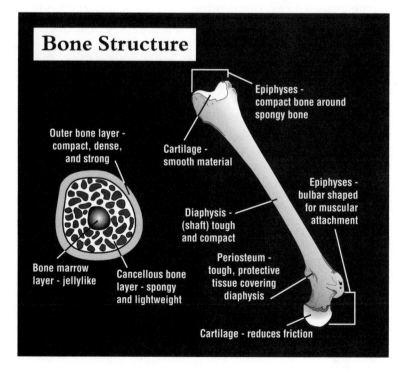

Bone Structure

Epiphyses - compact bone around spongy bone

Outer bone layer - compact, dense, and strong

Cartilage - smooth material

Epiphyses - bulbar shaped for muscular attachment

Diaphysis - (shaft) tough and compact

Bone marrow layer - jellylike

Cancellous bone layer - spongy and lightweight

Periosteum - tough, protective tissue covering diaphysis

Cartilage - reduces friction

epiphyses. Each epiphysis, with its bulbar shape, provides plenty of space for muscle attachment. An epiphysis consists of a thin layer of compact bone around a more loosely constructed area of spongy bone. Unlike the diaphysis, the epiphyses are not blanketed by the protective periosteum. Instead, they are covered by cartilage, a smooth material that reduces the friction between bones. In a young person, there is also a flat plate of cartilage in each epiphysis that allows the lengthwise growth of bones. After puberty, when growth is complete, these cartilaginous plates are turned to bone, leaving only a line to mark their previous locations.

Bone is living tissue, just like skin and blood. Unlike other tissues, some areas of bone have the ability to harden because they can hold deposits of minerals. Under the microscope, thin sections of hard bone look like mazes. This is because hard bones are riddled by millions of passageways that constitute paths for nerves and blood vessels, providing bone cells with nutrients and oxygen and affording channels of communication with the rest of the body.

Mature bone-forming cells, osteocytes, are located in hollow spaces called lacunae that are scattered throughout bone. Like tents around a campfire, lacunae are arranged in circular patterns around central shafts, or haversian canals. Haversian canals span the length of a bone, acting as conduits for the blood vessels and nerves that run from one end to the other. Tiny, spokelike tubes radiate from the central canals to connect individual cells to the bone's central supply lines.

Not Just for Halloween

A mature skeleton is basically made of two types of material—bone and cartilage. In embryos, however, the skeleton is primarily cartilage except for the skull, which also contains numerous strong, fibrous membranes. Cartilage is chemically similar to bone but is not as hard. Over time, nearly all soft cartilage and all fibrous membranes are replaced with hard bone so that by the time a baby reaches childhood most of the skeleton is bone. Throughout life, cartilage remains in areas such as the bridge of the nose, the ears, and the ends of ribs.

The replacement of cartilage and fibrous membranes with bone begins during fetal life. In this process, known as ossification, precursor bone-forming cells, or osteoblasts, produce a material called bone matrix, which completely covers the existing cartilage. Bone matrix acts like reinforced concrete for the skeleton. For a short while, the developing fetus has a cartilage skeleton covered with a bone skeleton. Eventually, the encircled cartilage is digested away and replaced by bone. By the time a child is born, much of its skeleton is bony.

When a baby is born, one area where ossification has not reached completion is the skull. The fibrous membranes, or fontanels, that connect the brain-covering plates to one another are not completely ossified at birth. The areas of membrane on a baby's skull are often referred to as soft spots. These membranes give a baby's head some flexibility and compressibility, characteristics that help the baby fit through the mother's rigid pelvic bones during the birthing process. Fontanels are gradually converted to bone during early infancy.

Between infancy and adulthood, bones grow in size. The relative sizes of bones change, also. At birth, the head is one-fourth of the body's total height. By adulthood, it makes up only one-eighth of total height. An infant's face is very small compared to the size of the skull, but with time the face size enlarges from one-eighth the size of the skull to one-half. With growth, the trunk becomes shorter relative to height, and the legs become longer.

As people age, bones continue to alter; they lose calcium, and their margins, or edges, change shape. Young people have very clean-cut, sharp bone margins, whereas elderly people have shaggy margins. This change is due to the development of projections called spurs and from the addition of extra bone, a change described as marginal lipping. These modifications contribute to the mobility problems experienced by many older people.

Cartilage begins to turn to bone while the fetus is still in the womb.

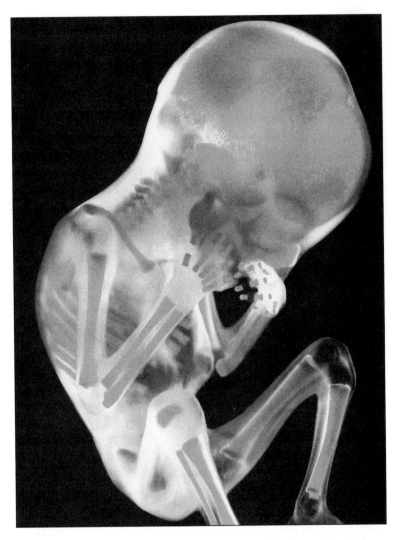

Although bone only grows from birth through adolescence, it is a living tissue that continually remodels itself all through life. Factors that stimulate remodeling are levels of calcium in the blood and the pull of gravity on muscles attached to bone.

The Consequence of Calcium

Calcium is one of the minerals responsible for forming the compounds that create hard bone. Calcium is also a player in other body functions, including nerve transmissions and muscle contractions. The concentration of calcium in the blood must remain constant for the body to function normally. Endocrine glands, which help regulate body functions, determine calcium levels. When blood calcium levels are low, small endocrine glands, the parathyroids, release a chemical called parathyroid hormone (PTH).

The presence of PTH activates osteoclasts, cells that are stored in the bone. Once triggered by hormones, osteoclasts set about releasing calcium into the blood. To do this, they destroy bone, breaking down the bone matrix to allow the calcium to enter the bloodstream. Thus, the presence of PTH raises the level of calcium in the blood by lowering its concentration in bones. On the other hand, when the concentration of calcium in the blood is high, another endocrine gland, the anterior pituitary, releases calcitonin. This hormone stimulates bone to absorb calcium, thereby building bone and reducing calcium concentration in the blood.

Even though blood calcium levels determine when bone is built or broken down, they do not decide where bone will be added or destroyed. Two physical forces, muscles tugging against bone and the pull of gravity, control where bone is formed. Exercises like walking or weight lifting cause stress as muscles pull on bone, and bone responds by creating new bone at the stress points where muscles attach. Therefore, much of the bone remodeling that occurs during life is related to use, because bones become thicker in areas where large muscles attach. At attachment sites, osteoblasts deposit new layers of bone matrix. The cells themselves become trapped in the sticky matrix they exude, and there they mature into osteocytes, forming areas of new bone. On the other hand, lack of movement also remodels bone. People who are paralyzed or physically unable to move for other reasons lose bone mass because their muscles are not working against their bones. And astronauts traveling in space, where there is no gravity, face the same problem; they must perform regular exercises to keep their bones strong.

At the Top of the Long Skeleton

The longitudinal, or "long" skeleton, comprises the bones of the head and trunk. These bones, also called axial bones, are the skull, the vertebral column, and the ribs. The top-most part of the human body, the skull, contains bones of two types: cranial and facial. The flat bones of the cranium surround and protect the brain. Facial bones support the muscles of the face and hold the eyes in front of the head. The only movable bone in the skull is the lower jawbone, or mandible, which is attached to the rest of the skull with a movable joint. All the other bones are attached to one another at fixed, or stationary, joints called sutures. The movable bone is also the largest and strongest bone of the face and is the bone that holds the lower teeth. The upper teeth are found in the two maxillae, or maxillary bones, which fuse to form the upper jaw.

Although not technically part of the skull, the hyoid bone is located near the mandible. The hyoid is unusual because it is the only bone in the body that does not articulate to, or join, another bone. It is held in place in the midneck, direct-ly above the larynx, by several muscles.

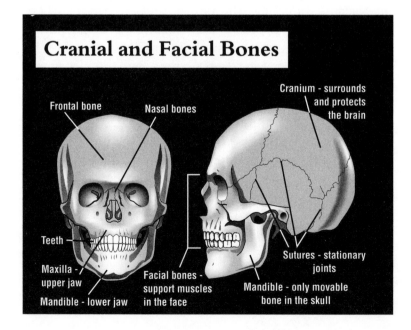

Cranial and Facial Bones

Frontal bone

Nasal bones

Cranium - surrounds and protects the brain

Teeth

Maxilla - upper jaw

Mandible - lower jaw

Facial bones - support muscles in the face

Sutures - stationary joints

Mandible - only movable bone in the skull

The Rest of the Long Skeleton

Below the skull is the vertebral column, or spine, which extends down to the pelvis. The spine carries over two dozen irregularly shaped bones that are attached to one another by ligaments to form a flexible, S-shaped curve. The spinal cord, a large trunk of delicate nerve fibers, runs through the central cavity of these bones or vertebrae.

Vertebrae are not stacked one on top of another like building blocks. Instead they are separated by pads of cartilage called intervertebral disks. Disks prevent vertebrae from rubbing against one another. They have high water content, so they are spongy and compressible, serving as good shock absorbers for the spine. As one ages, disks lose water and become harder and thinner.

All vertebrae resemble one another, yet each has its own distinctive features. Most are short and rounded, with processes, or extensions, where muscles attach. Many vertebrae also have points on them where they connect to ribs. The curved shape of the overall spine is an adaptation that increases its carrying strength. At birth, the spine has a rounded, or convex, shape from head to tailbone. Later, as the child sits and stands, the familiar S-shape develops.

The seven vertebrae located at the base of the skull and in the neck are cervical vertebrae. The first of these is called the atlas because it has the role of holding up the head, much like the mythical giant Atlas held up the world. The second vertebra is the axis, which serves as a pivot to allow the head to tilt forward and back. The remaining five bones complete the structure of the neck.

Vertebrae of the spine are divided into four groups: thoracic, lumbar, sacral, and coccygeal. Twelve thoracic vertebrae support the upper back, and four lumbar vertebrae form the lower back. The sacrum, which is made from the fusion of five vertebrae, and the coccyx, or tailbone, which is created by the fusion of four small vertebrae, complete the spine.

Along with the ribs and sternum, the thoracic vertebrae form the thorax, the bony cage that encloses the heart and lungs. Ribs are long, curved bones that extend from the

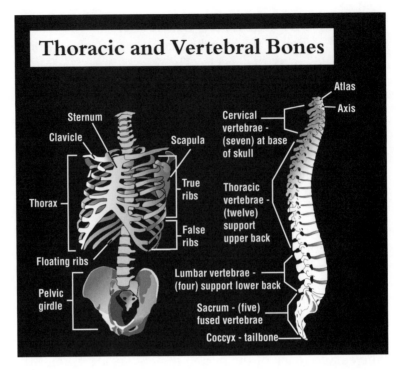

Thoracic and Vertebral Bones

spine to the front of the body. The sternum, or breastbone, attaches to some of the ribs in the front of the chest. Together, these bones surround and protect the heart and lungs as well as large blood vessels. Humans, both male and female, have twelve pairs of ribs. The first seven pairs, the true ribs, are attached to the sternum by cartilage. The next five pairs are called false ribs; these pairs attach indirectly. The last two pairs, called floating ribs, do not attach to the sternum at all.

The Appendicular Skeleton

The bones that make up the appendicular skeleton are found in the shoulder girdles and the pelvic girdle, the bony belts that make up these areas. Each shoulder girdle is made of two bones, the clavicle and the scapula. The clavicle, or collarbone, is long, slender, and curved. Its job is to act as a brace that holds the arm away from the top part of the thorax. The scapula, or shoulder blade, is a flattened bone with a triangular shape. Not directly attached to the axial skeleton, it is held loosely in place by muscles of the back so that it can slide back and forth as those muscles move.

Each upper limb contains thirty-two individual bones. The upper arm is made of one bone, the humerus, which has a typical long bone shape and form. The lower arm, or forearm, contains two bones, the radius and ulna. The radius is on the thumb side when the hands are held facing forward. The other twenty-nine bones of the upper limb are found in each hand, and they are of three basic types: wrist bones are carpals, palm bones are metacarpals, and finger bones are phalanges. Each finger has three phalanges.

Whereas the upper body has both a right and left shoulder girdle and a right and left arm, the lower body has one pelvic girdle and a right and left leg. The pelvic girdle is really two structures fused into one. Each contains a coxal, or hipbone, which is made of part of the sacrum and part of the coccyx. All of the bones of the pelvic girdle are large and heavy because they have the responsibility of bearing the weight of the entire upper body. They also house and protect the reproductive organs, bladder, and part of the intestine. In general, the pelvic girdle has a bowl shape with a large opening in the center. Male and female pelvises bear some distinctions related to function. The female pelvis is shallower and the bones lighter and thinner than the male pelvis. The opening in the middle of the female pelvis, the inlet, is larger and more circular than that of the male pelvis. In females, a baby must travel through the inlet during birth, and the opening must be big enough to accommodate the baby's head.

Like the upper arm, the upper leg contains only one bone, the femur. This thighbone is the heaviest and strongest bone in the body. It is a typical long bone with a large, ball-like head that fits into the pelvic cavity. The lower leg contains two bones, the tibia and fibula. Of the two, the tibia, or shinbone, is larger and stronger. The tibia joins the femur to form a knee joint. A small bone, the patella, or knee-cap, protects the joint. Even though the fibula lies alongside the tibia, it is not part of the knee joint. This thin bone is found deeper within the leg than the tibia, and it forms part of the outer ankle.

The foot has the job of supporting the entire body. It also works as a lever to allow forward motion. The basic structure of a foot includes the ankle, sole, and toes. Seven tarsals make up the ankle. The largest and most prominent two are the calcaneus, or heel bone, and the talus, located between the tibia and calcaneus. Five metatarsals form the sole of the foot, and fourteen phalanges make up the toes. Like fingers, each toe contains three bones.

Skeletal Attributes of Athletes

In all movement, the skeletal and muscular systems work hand in hand. Athletes, people who push their bodies to their physical limits, work constantly to improve the conditions of these body systems. The muscular system can be trained to work harder and faster. The skeletal system, on the other hand, is fairly fixed and cannot be improved. However, exercise stimulates the body to replace old bone with new, adding strength to bone structure.

The skeletal system plays a role in determining a person's overall suitability for a sport. Much research has been dedicated to determining ideal bone and skeletal system dimensions for each sport. The science of bones in sports is called kinanthropometrics. Research shows that, in general, three considerations affect an athlete's suitability for a sport: overall size, proportions of the skeleton, and size of some critical bones.

Overall size, or total body height, is rarely a limiting factor. A young person who reaches an overall size of five and one-half feet may not be best suited to professional basketball but might excel as a swimmer or long-distance runner. However, in most sports, the proportioning of an athlete's skeleton is a bigger consideration than overall size. Proportion refers to the size of the upper body, or trunk, relative to the lower body, or legs. Skeletal proportion helps determine one's center of gravity and affects balance, an important consideration in sports. The longer the upper

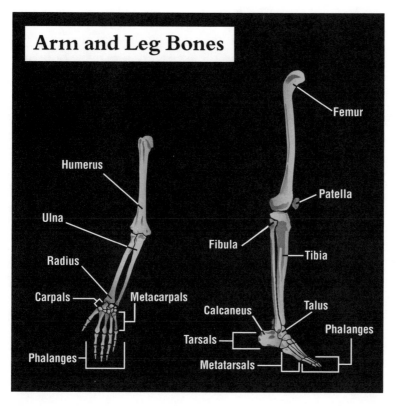

Arm and Leg Bones

Femur

Humerus

Patella

Ulna

Fibula

Tibia

Radius

Carpals

Metacarpals

Calcaneus

Talus

Phalanges

Tarsals

Phalanges

Metatarsals

body in proportion to the lower body, the lower the center of gravity. Runners need a high center of gravity for fluid movement of the legs during races. Football players who fill the position of fullback need a low center of gravity to help maintain their balance when being tackled.

Boning Up

Everyone, athlete and nonathlete alike, has the same basic body plan. In this plan, bones form the skeletal framework. Without a skeleton, the body would be a shapeless mass of tissue. Besides giving support, bones protect delicate organs, store fat and minerals, and serve as sites where new cells are made.

Bones are strong, stiff structures. For the body to be flexible, individual bones are joined at points called joints. Here, they come together in a way that allows one bone to move and the other to remain stationary. Muscles provide the power for moving bones, thus creating motions as varied as playing the piano and jumping on a trampoline.

Of all the body systems, the skeletal system is the only one that cannot be trained to improve. Unlike muscle, the skeleton does not increase in size because of exercise. However, work and motion stimulate new bone tissues to replace old ones, so bones can grow stronger.

2 | The Muscular System

Bones, the body's movable supports, make motion possible. However, these rigid tissues cannot move themselves; something must pull them. That something is muscle. Bones provide the framework against which muscles can work. Together, bones and muscles enable the body to move in thousands of ways.

Muscles are bulky tissues that cover the skeleton and provide the body with its overall shape. In many cases, the outlines of individual muscles can be seen under the skin. The name *muscle* comes from the Latin word *mus*, which means "mouse," because ancients thought that rippling muscles looked like mice running beneath the skin.

Almost all of the body's 650 different muscles are constantly at work. The expression of nearly all thoughts depends on movement. Even though muscles are essential for movement, they also have other important jobs. Muscles are constantly performing such tasks as focusing the eyes, lifting the lungs during inhalation, and swallowing food. Muscles also keep the heart beating, food moving along the digestive tract, and blood flowing through vessels.

Muscles are tissues that have the unique ability to contract. Based on their structure, muscles are classified into three types: skeletal, smooth, and cardiac. Most of the muscle in the body is skeletal. In fact, the volume of skeletal muscle is so great that it makes up about one-half of the total body weight. As its name implies, skeletal muscle attaches to the skeleton. By pulling bone in one direction or the other, skeletal muscle causes the body to move.

The Skeleton's Partner

Skeletal muscle has a few nicknames, like striated muscle and voluntary muscle. The term *striated* describes its striped appearance under the microscope. Skeletal muscle is also called voluntary because much of the body's skeletal muscle can be controlled by will or mind. When a person lifts a foot to kick a ball, the muscles that respond are skeletal muscles. Without skeletal muscles, a person could not reach for a glass of water or lean over to tie a shoe. Skeletal muscle is also responsible for movements such as walking, stretching, swimming, scratching, chewing, jogging, and lifting. Even so, there are some skeletal muscles that are involved in automatic or reflex motions; these types of movement do not require conscious thought.

A magnified cross section clearly shows the striated, or striped, delineations in muscle tissue.

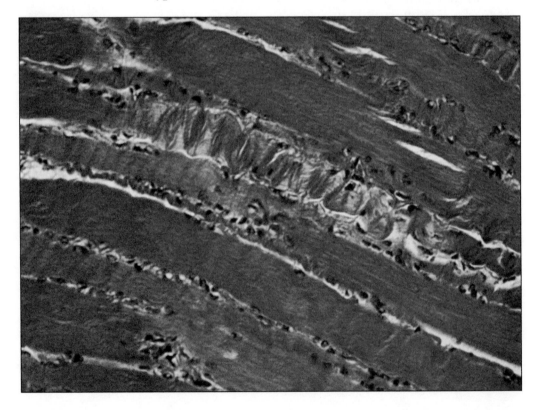

Skeletal muscle, a bulky yet somewhat delicate tissue, is heavily packaged. Each muscle is wrapped in a sheath of strong connective tissue, and groups of sheathed muscles are bound together by coarse fibers called fascicles. Sets of fascicle-covered muscles are enclosed in a tough outer coat of tissue that merges into tendons, the fibers that attach muscles to bones, cartilage, or other connective tissue. Tendons are stronger than muscle but not as strong as bone. Because tendons are so tough, they can reach over the rough ends of bones at joints without suffering any damage.

Macho Muscle Cells

A skeletal muscle is made of thousands of individual muscle cells. All body cells, including those in muscles, nerve tissue, and skin, have the same basic design. A cell membrane wraps around and contains the cytoplasm, a living, jellylike material in the cell. The job of a cell membrane is to regulate what enters and leaves the cell. Tiny pores can be opened and closed to allow materials to travel through the membrane. Within the cytoplasm is a command post, or nucleus, which contains genetic information and controls cellular activities. Several organelles, little organlike structures, are scattered through the cytoplasm.

One of these organelles, the tubular-shaped endoplasmic reticulum, extends through much of the cytoplasm. It provides a conduit from the nucleus to other organelles. All cells also contain hundreds of mitochondria, small organelles that convert glucose into energy. Other structures in cells include storage sacs called vacuoles, ribosomes that make proteins, and Golgi bodies, which package proteins for export.

Muscle cells are uniquely specialized for their job of contracting. Each muscle cell is a giant compared to other body cells. Muscle cells are both larger and longer than other cell types, and instead of one nucleus, they contain several scattered throughout the cytoplasm. A muscle cell is enclosed by its sarcolemma, a strong covering made of a cell membrane plus a protective outer coat. The cytoplasm, called sarcoplasm, contains the typical organelles, but some are

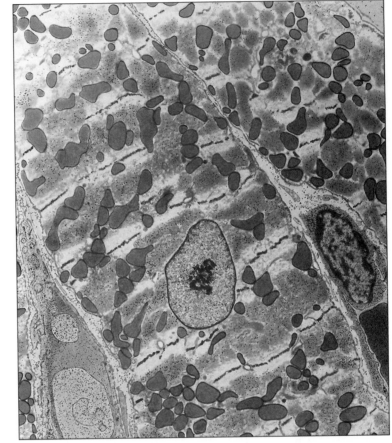

The circular nucleus (center) of a muscle cell is surrounded by many mitochondria clusters that fuel the cell's activity.

customized for their functions in muscle. For example, the endoplasmic reticulum is modified into a much larger form and is called the sarcoplastic reticulum. Because muscle cells use more energy than most other cell types, they contain exceptionally large numbers of mitochondria.

Energy to Burn

Every cell in the body must have energy to stay alive and function. Cells have several energy-producing strategies to ensure that a supply is always available. They keep a small amount of energy on hand in a ready-to-use form, plus they have some stored in an easily accessible form. Once these supplies are used up, cells must make additional energy.

In cells, a molecule called adenosine triphosphate, or ATP, stores energy until it is needed. Muscle cells always have a small supply of ATP on hand, enough to work at maximum power for about three seconds. This ATP enables muscles to respond immediately to stimuli. Muscles also contain creatine phosphate, a compound that can quickly generate additional ATP. The ATP from creatine phosphate can keep up maximum power for another five seconds. Therefore, the two energy sources that are immediately available for a muscle are the ready-to-use ATP and the ATP made from creatine phosphate.

When creatine phosphate is consumed, cells begin to break down, or burn, glucose for energy. Some glucose is present in cells in a stored form called glycogen. Other glucose molecules, the products of digestion, are delivered to cells by the blood as they become available.

Glucose can be quickly converted to energy, or metabolized, as long as there is plenty of oxygen available. Glucose metabolism is similar to wood burning. Glucose and wood are both forms of fuel, and their breakdown works best when oxygen is abundant. The metabolism of glucose in the presence of oxygen is called aerobic respiration. It is a very efficient process that yields a lot of energy. The oxygen that cells use in aerobic respiration originates in the lungs and is delivered to individual cells by the bloodstream.

If a muscle is working very hard, as it does during exercise, the lungs and blood may not be able to supply oxygen fast enough to maintain the aerobic breakdown of glucose. When this happens, muscle cells are forced to rely on a less efficient mechanism to keep going: the anaerobic breakdown of glucose. Like a fire that is smoldering, the anaerobic metabolism of glucose produces much smaller quantities of energy. During anaerobic metabolism, a by-product called lactic acid is created. Accumulation of lactic acid can interfere with a muscle's ability to work.

Like machines, cells must generate energy to perform work; however, the production of energy for work is not 100 percent efficient. Both cells and machines lose much of their energy as heat. Seventy-five percent of the energy produced in a cell is converted to heat energy, leaving only 25 percent to work in the cell. During normal day-to-day activities, the heat is carried to other tissues by the blood to help maintain body temperature. However, when muscle cells are extremely active, they produce more heat than the body needs, creating the need to cool the body by mechanisms such as sweating.

Tighten Up

Since muscle cells have elongated shapes, they are often described as fibers. A muscle fiber is made up of thin, elastic units called myofibrils. Like a rubber band, myofibrils have a stretchy quality to them that allows expansion and contraction. The stretchability of an individual myofibril is due to the two types of protein filaments within it, myosin and actin. These proteins also make contraction possible.

Within a muscle fiber, strands of myosin and actin proteins lie in precise patterns. The dark, thick strands of myosin contrast vividly with the pale, thin threads of actin. The alternating arrangement of these two different kinds of fibers creates the light and dark bands, the striations, that are characteristic of skeletal muscle. The light actin bands have a midband line running through them called the Z line. The dark bands of myosin contain a similar, but paler, midline called the H zone. The segment of muscle between two Z lines, a sarcomere, acts as a tiny contractile unit.

Within a sarcomere, actin and myosin overlap in two areas. In these areas of overlap, the two protein fibers lie side by side. Myosin fibers have abundant supplies of an enzyme that helps generate ATP, and they are studded with globular knobs called cross fibers that stick out in all directions. Cross fibers play a critical role in the contraction process by forming links with strands of actin. These links allow myosin cross fibers to "walk" up the length of actin fibers, pulling the two strands closer together, contracting or shortening the muscle.

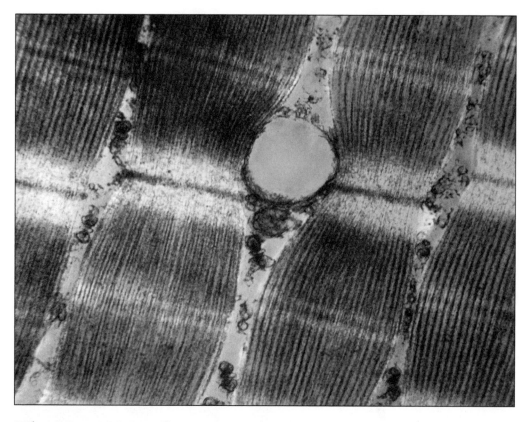

The Nerve-Muscle Connection

Muscles take their orders from the nervous system. Specifically, the brain sends a signal to a muscle telling it to contract or relax. Each muscle fiber receives its signals from one nerve called a motor neuron. Motor neurons start in the brain and extend down the spinal cord; then each one exits to a point very near its assigned muscle fiber. The neuron does not make direct contact with the muscle, however; there is a microscopic gap between the nerve and the muscle fiber.

The signals carried by motor neurons exist in the form of electrical impulses. After an impulse has successfully navigated the length of a motor neuron, it must cross the gap to reach the muscle. To accomplish this, neurons call on a sophisticated transport system. The muscle end of a neuron is rich in tiny sacs that contain chemicals called neurotransmitters. When an electrical impulse reaches the end of a

Characteristic of skeletal muscle, a magnified image shows a striated pattern in the muscle fiber.

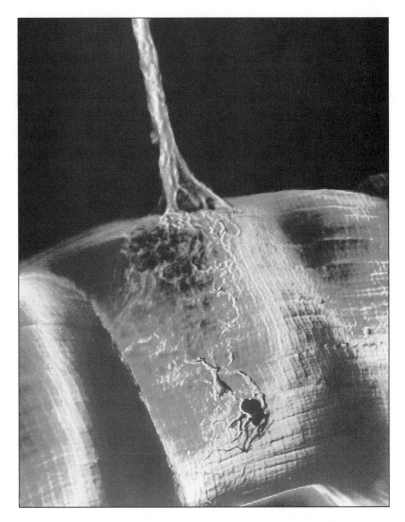

nerve, it stimulates these sacs to open, releasing their contents. Neurotransmitters flow across the gap between the
nerve and muscle fiber, carrying the stimulus to the muscle
fiber. The muscle fiber contracts when the neurotransmitters reach it, and thus motion occurs without the nerve itself
ever touching the muscle.

When examined closely, a contraction is a multistage
event that depends on the electrical impulse plus the movement of minerals in and out of muscle cells. Each step of the
process requires energy, which is supplied in the form of
ATP. When an electrical impulse stimulates a cell, it opens

the pores in its membrane, allowing electrically charged particles of sodium to flow into the cell. The presence inside the cell of these charged particles of sodium stimulates the sarcoplasmic reticulum to release calcium ions. Calcium ions cause the formation of links between actin and myosin filaments. Once connected, the two fibers can slide together, contracting the muscle. After a fraction of a second, calcium returns to the sarcoplasmic reticulum, where it stays until the next electrical impulse comes along. Without calcium, linkages between actin and myosin are broken, and the muscle relaxes.

Sometimes muscles cramp, or contract painfully, without being able to relax. Cramps occur when ATP supplies are too low to break the links between actin and myosin. If the body runs completely out of ATP, death occurs. Several hours after death, calcium leaks out of cell structures, causing all the muscles in the body to contract, a condition called rigor mortis. Without any ATP to return calcium to the sarcoplasmic reticulum, the cross bridges between actin and myosin cannot be broken and the contraction cannot end. Therefore, rigor mortis continues until the actin and myosin proteins begin to decompose, about fifteen to twenty-five hours after death.

Building Bigger Bodies

Exercise puts an additional burden on the body's muscular and skeletal systems, causing them to stretch their capabilities. Moderate exercise is an excellent way to keep both systems in optimal health, but extreme exercise can push them to perform at their limits. During any type of competition, an athlete depends on the strength and power of muscles. The size of a muscle establishes its strength, and the amount of work it can do determines its power.

The basic size of a muscle is dictated by heredity but is subject to levels of testosterone in the body. Testosterone is a sex hormone that influences growth and development; it is found in much larger quantities in males than females.

Testosterone stimulates the production of new tissue, like muscle, from protein. A man with normal levels of testosterone has muscles that are 40 percent larger than those of a woman with typical testosterone levels for a female.

Training or exercise can cause muscles to increase in size, or hypertrophy, by an additional 30 to 60 percent. When a muscle gets larger, the diameter of each of its individual fibers enlarges. Within a muscle fiber, exercise causes some specific, measurable changes, such as increases in the number of myofibrils, increases in the levels of chemicals that assist energy production in mitochondria, increases in the quantity of creatine phosphate, and increases in the amount of stored glycogen. All together, these changes improve the rate, as well as the efficiency, of processes within muscle cells.

Moving Muscles

Muscles are able to create movement because they treat bones as levers. A lever is a device used to move something. To be effective, a lever must be fixed at one end, a point called the fulcrum. The other, movable end can then be used to push against a resistance. In the body, the fulcrum end of a bone is attached to another bone, while the other end of that bone is free to move. One or more muscles pull the movable end of the bone, causing motion.

The part of the muscle attached to the fulcrum is called the origin. The other end, on the movable part of the bone, is the insertion. Usually, the end of the muscle that is closest to the center of the body is the origin, and the end furthest away is the insertion. When a muscle contracts, the insertion is pulled toward the origin.

Some muscles have more than one point of origin or insertion. For example, the biceps, whose name means "two heads," has two origins. The two heads of a biceps muscle originate in the shoulder girdle; the muscle has one insertion in the radius of the forearm. The lower arm is moved by contracting the biceps muscle. In this movement, the radius is the lever and the elbow serves as the fulcrum.

Most types of movement require more than one muscle, so muscles usually work in groups. The relationship of pairs of muscles involved in movement can be observed by watching the body move. For example, when the arm is lifted to the side, the muscle on top of the shoulder, the deltoid, contracts. Since the deltoid is responsible for this move, it is called a prime mover. However, other muscles are moving, too, and these muscles, which contract and assist the prime mover, are called synergists.

The prime mover and synergists have counterparts called antagonists. As the name implies, antagonists resist a prime mover's action and cause movement in the opposite direction. For example, the antagonist to the prime mover that raises the arm is the muscle that lowers the arm. If a prime mover and its antagonist contract at the same time, all of the muscles remain rigid and no motion occurs. Therefore, for body movements to occur, a prime mover must relax when its antagonist contracts, and vice versa. The brain is in charge of coordinating the relaxation of some muscles and the contraction of others so that smooth, fluid motion is possible.

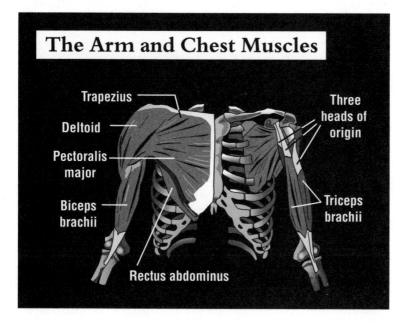

The Arm and Chest Muscles

Trapezius

Deltoid

Pectoralis major

Biceps brachii

Three heads of origin

Triceps brachii

Rectus abdominus

Muscle Up

The 650 skeletal muscles found in the body are often studied in groups. Muscles of the head are usually separated into two sets: facial muscles and muscles used for chewing. Most facial muscles have a unique quality; instead of attaching to bone like almost all other muscles, they attach to skin. Therefore, when facial muscles contract, they pull on the skin of the face, creating thousands of expressions such as smiles, frowns, grimaces, sneers, and grins. The zygomaticus, or smiling muscle, runs from the corner of the mouth to the cheekbone. When it contracts, it pulls the corners of the lips upward. The orbicularis oris, the kissing muscle, wraps around the mouth and permits the lips to pucker. All together there are 60 muscles in the face; 20 of them are used to smile and 40 to frown.

Chewing is primarily controlled by two large muscles, the masseter and the temporalis. The masseter begins below the eye and runs down the cheek, covering the mandible, or jawbone. It closes the jaw by bringing the mandible up to meet the unmoving maxilla. The temporalis is in front of and above the ear; it works with the masseter to close the jaw.

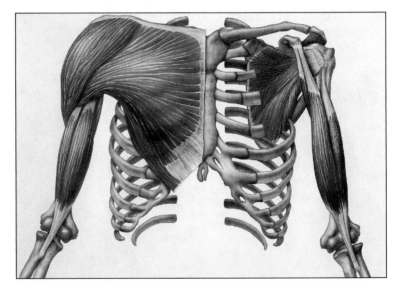

A drawing depicts the sternum and rib cage, and the surrounding trunk muscles that are responsible for arm movement.

Neck muscles, which are shaped like straps, work with muscles on the trunk to support and move the head and the shoulder girdle. Trunk muscles also move the vertebral column, the ribs, and the arms. The pectoralis major is a large, fan-shaped muscle on each side of the upper chest. The two muscles are nicknamed the pectorals, or pecs. At puberty, the pecs of young boys often begin to develop and become noticeable. Pecs can also be seen in athletes and in bodybuilders. The musculature in the abdomen creates part of the body wall, supporting the internal organs. The rectus abdominus, the abdominal muscles, or abs, start beneath the rib cage and cover the stomach. Fibers of each muscle run in different directions, so the abs are very strong even though they are not extremely thick.

The trapezius muscles originate at the base of the skull and along the vertebral column and then extend to the midshoulder, on either side of the spine, to insert in the scapula and clavicle. When viewed together, the trapezius muscles form a diamond shape. They lift, lower, and tighten the scapulas, as well as hold them in place. A large, triangular muscle, the deltoid, begins at the trapezius and covers each shoulder. Because it is so big, the deltoid is a favorite site for medical injections that must be given intramuscularly. The deltoids move the shoulders in all directions and help lift the arms.

When asked to "make a muscle," most people tighten and display the biceps brachii in the forearm. The triceps brachii, on the back of the arm, is a long muscle that has three heads of origins. This muscle is the prime mover of elbow extension and antagonist of the biceps. The triceps is sometimes called the boxer's muscle because it can deliver a straight-arm punch.

The largest muscles are found in the lower body. The big muscle that covers the hip is the gluteus maximus. The four bulky muscles on the front of the thigh are called the quadriceps, or quads. These make it possible to walk, run, kick, and ride a bike. The hamstring group, made of three large muscles, covers the back of the thigh. The name comes from the fact that butchers use these muscles to hang slabs of meat called hams for smoking. In the lower leg, the gastrocnemius, or "toe dancer's" muscle, is a two-part structure that forms the curve of the calf.

Beating and Squeezing

The body's internal organs contain no skeletal muscle. Rather, movement in organs is provided by specialized muscles that differ significantly from skeletal muscles in structure and function. Smooth muscle makes up the walls of organs like the stomach, intestine, and bladder. Since these muscles contract without conscious control, they are also described as involuntary. Involuntary muscles control such functions as digestion of food and movement of blood through vessels.

In some organs, smooth muscle plays roles in both voluntary and involuntary behavior. For example, within the bladder and the rectum, smooth muscles contract without conscious thought to hold their contents in place. However, the brain can override these muscles and consciously cause them to relax, a mechanism that enables people to plan their trips to the bathroom. On the other hand, there are situations that cause smooth muscles to stop doing their jobs. When someone is extremely frightened, the muscles in the bladder may suddenly relax, releasing their watery contents.

Smooth and striated muscles have some important differences. Unlike their skeletal cousins, smooth muscles are not striated. Each cell is long and pointed on each end, with a single nucleus, unlike the multinucleated skeletal muscles. Smooth muscles are usually arranged in pairs of layers, one lying circularly and the other longitudinally. As the layers contract and relax, they change the shape of the organ, squeezing it. Whereas striated muscle can move quickly if necessary, the actions of smooth muscles are slow and steady.

Cardiac muscle, found only in the heart, is different from both skeletal and smooth muscle: It is striated and involuntary. Cardiac muscle contracts strongly and rhythmically,

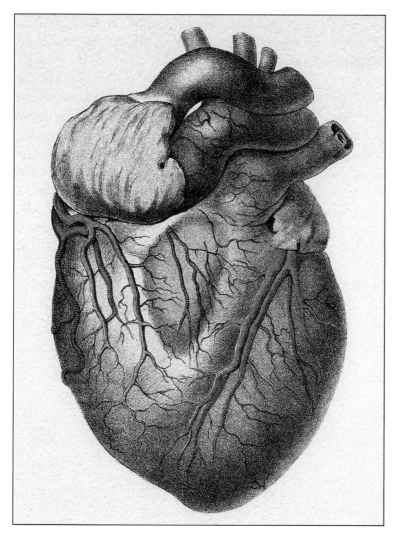

The heart is perhaps the most important muscle in the body. It pumps life-giving blood to muscles, bones, and organs.

sending blood through the body in powerful surges. The multinucleated cells in cardiac muscle are joined end to end, a characteristic that lets the electrical current that creates heart rhythm flow quickly from cell to cell.

The Muscle Story

Muscles, tissues that have the ability to contract, are often associated with strength. However, everyone, the weak and the strong, has muscles; some people have more prominent muscles than others. Muscles make up almost half of a person's body mass, and they give the body its shape. Working with the skeletal system, muscles make it possible to move.

Skeletal muscle is the type that lifts the arms, turns the head, and snaps the fingers. Designed to work hard for short periods of time, much of the body's skeletal muscle is under voluntary control. Skeletal muscle appears to be striated because of the way its fibers are organized. Smooth muscle, which makes up the wall of blood vessels and organs like the stomach and bladder, does not have any striations and is not under voluntary control. It is responsible for the slow, steady contractions that squeeze blood along vessels, move food through the digestive system, and hold urine in the bladder. Cardiac muscle, specialized for constant, strong contractions, is also involuntary. However, unlike smooth muscle, it has prominent striations formed from bands of fibers. Cardiac muscle is responsible for pumping blood through the body.

3 | The Joints of the Body

Working as a team, bones and muscles enable humans to walk, run, grasp, and sit. Since bones are rigid and do not have the ability to bend, one might wonder how they could function in activities of so many kinds. The answer to that question is found in the body's sixty-eight joints. A joint is an area where two bones come together, or articulate. Without joints, movement would be so stiff that everyone would walk like a robot.

Although most humans are able to move, not all people have the same range of motion. Some people are very flexible, either because they have stretched their muscles through exercises or because they are born that way. People who can maneuver their body with extreme flexibility are considered to have hypermobile joints and may be described as double-jointed. Niccolo Paganini, a virtuoso violinist of the nineteenth century, is one of the first recorded cases of hypermobility. At Paganini's concerts, the audience was stunned by the flexibility of his fingers on the violin. Paganini had such loose joints that he could bend his left thumb backward so that it touched the back of his hand as his fingers raced across the strings. Paginini's incredible flexibility may have contributed to his exceptional skill as a violinist.

Houdini, the great escape artist, was another famous double-jointed person. He used his flexibility to escape from chains or ropes that bound him. Houdini's illusions of magic often put him in great personal danger, and he depended on his ability to dislocate his joints, or take his bones out of their normal joint positions, to escape. He practiced this technique until he could do it easily.

Moving on Up

Movement, whether normal or hypermobile, is a characteristic shared by most animals. Many mammals, the group containing humans and the animals to which they are most closely related, are born with the ability to stand and walk a few moments after birth. However, humans do not develop the ability to move from one place to another for several months after they are born. At the age of four months, most children begin to pull up into a standing position, and by nine months many children can crawl. As the age of a child increases, so do the powers of locomotion. Somewhere between twelve and eighteen months of age, most children learn to walk, and by the time they are two years old many can move about at a slow trot. By three years of age, many children are beginning to develop the ability to run, and by four years of age they can hop.

Humans can perform an astonishing variety of movements. Joints work with muscles and bones to permit a foot to pivot a ballerina on the tips of the toes or a soccer player to kick a ball across the field. The versatility of human motion is due to the number and types of joints in the body. Not all joints are the same. The structure of a joint determines how much motion it will allow as well as the direction of movement. Joints are categorized in two different ways: by their anatomical structure or by the degree of movement that they allow. The structural types of joints are fibrous, cartilaginous, and synovial. Joint categories based on movement are immovable, slightly movable, or freely movable.

What Kind of Joint Is This?

Joints exist in a variety of shapes and sizes. Each is especially designed to accommodate movement in the body part that it serves. Except for the hyoid bone in the neck, every bone in the human body forms a joint with at least one other bone. All joints, no matter what their job, share some characteristics in common. The two bones of a joint, for example, are always connected by either fibrous tissue or cartilage.

The group of joints that are described as immovable are held together with dense mats of fibrous connective tissue: strong fibers that knit the adjoining bone surfaces close together. Immovable joints are bound so closely by fibrous tissue that no space, or joint cavity, exists between the two bones. The most common kind of immovable joint is the suture, the type of joint that connects the forty bony plates of the skull. In a developing fetus, the skull sutures are held loosely together, a feature that makes the infant's head somewhat flexible, enabling it to pass through the narrow birth canal. After birth, the loose connections between these cranial plates gradually begin to harden, and the bony areas fuse. By adulthood, the cranial plates have ossified into a solid, protective enclosure for the brain. Suture joints are also located between the radius and ulna of the arm, between the tibia and fibula of the leg, and between the root of a tooth and the jawbone.

In joints that are considered to be slightly movable, the two bones are bound together with cartilage, a flexible, white, elastic tissue. Cartilaginous joints, like fibrous ones, lack a joint cavity; that is, there is only minimal space between the articulating bones. The cartilage connections at these points hold the bones closely together, but not quite as tightly as the fibrous tissue in immovable joints. Cartilaginous joints do allow a small amount of movement. For example, the spine can bend and twist because vertebrae are connected to each other by cartilaginous joints. The regions of cartilage between each pair of vertebrae are described as disks. Every disk has an outer rim made of tough cartilage surrounding a pulpy, elastic core. These cartilage pads help absorb shock to the spine caused by walking and assist in equalizing pressure along the back as the body moves. Disks can be damaged by time or by physical injury.

An MRI scan shows a side view of a slipped disk (pointed, lower right) penetrating the spinal cord beside it (lighter, lengthwise strip). The result is severe pain.

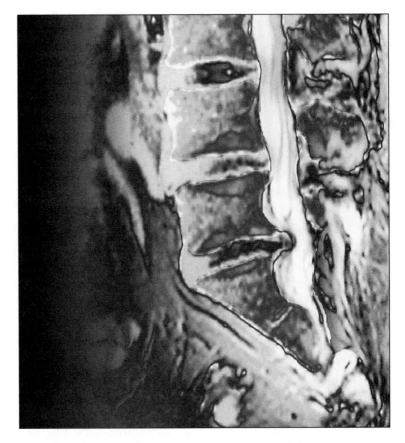

As a person ages, the disks can lose some of their resiliency, making bending more difficult and causing some back discomfort. A sudden trauma to disks can compress them, sending fragments of bone protruding into the spinal canal. These jutting pieces can cause severe pain and are often referred to as slipped or herniated disks.

The bones of the ribs and the sternum also have cartilaginous joints to accommodate expansion of the chest cavity during inhalation. Another location in the body where slight movement is necessary is at the pubic symphysis, located between the two pubic bones. During childbirth, the somewhat movable pubic joint allows the bones to widen, aiding the passage of the baby through the woman's pelvis. Cartilaginous joints are also found between the epiphyses of the long bones in adults and between the diaphyses in bones of children and teenagers. When the growth process is complete at adulthood, bone tissue has replaced the fibrous cartilage in these connections.

The types of joints that permit the greatest amount of movement are called freely movable, or synovial, joints. These are responsible for the flexibility of areas like the knee, shoulder, wrist, and ankle. Synovial joints are the most complex, as well as the most numerous, type of joints in the human body. There are many kinds of synovial joints, and each allows a different range of motion.

Up Close and Personal in a Synovial Joint

All synovial joints contain the same basic components: a joint capsule, a synovial membrane, articulating cartilage, a joint cavity, and ligaments. A joint capsule is made of an extension of the periosteum, or protective outer coating, of each bone in the joint. The capsule, which is a tough fibrous tissue, forms an outer casing around the ends of the bones, holding them in place. The synovial joint, inside the joint capsule, is a thin layer of cartilage; it forms an inner cover that cushions the ends of the bones. The inside surface of the joint capsule has a slippery, moist surface called the synovial membrane, which secretes a thick liquid. This synovial fluid has two important functions. It lubricates the joint, very much like grease on two meshing gears, permitting the parts to work together without friction. The fluid also provides tissues in the joint with oxygen and nutrients, an essential function since the cartilage at the end of bones cannot supply blood directly. The synovial fluid is contained in the joint cavity, an open area between the adjoining bones. No tissue grows in this space so that the bones can move freely around each other without friction. In some joints, such as those found in the shoulder, the synovial fluid is contained in special membranous sacs called bursae that help cushion muscles and tendons, preventing them from rubbing against bones.

The supportive tissues, ligaments, and tendons in and around a joint play vital roles in movement. Ligaments are strong, cordlike bands of fibrous tissue that attach bones firmly together. These bands are so strong that they are largely responsible for holding the two bones in their correct positions in the joint. Ligaments will stretch, much like rubber bands, and this elasticity helps bones move smoothly. There is a limit to how far a ligament can extend, however. If a movement stretches a ligament past its normal limit, it will be damaged or torn. A sprain occurs when a ligament is stretched so much that it completely or partially tears. When a joint receives a hard blow, the ligaments stretch as far as possible and then tear if the impact is more than the fibers can withstand. It is not unusual for ligaments to be torn in high-impact sports such as football and rugby. Sports-related ligament tears are common in the joints of the ankles and knees. Ligaments that are torn will not heal without treatment, and until the ligament is restored, the joint is unstable and susceptible to further injury.

No less important than ligaments in smooth locomotion is cartilage. Like a supersponge, this connective tissue absorbs large quantities of synovial fluid. When the joint is at rest, cartilage fills to capacity with the fluid. Once a per-

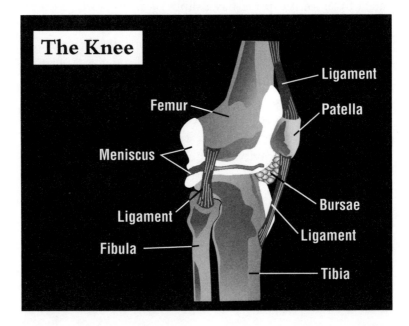

The Knee

Ligament

Femur

Patella

Meniscus

Bursae

Ligament

Ligament

Fibula

Tibia

son begins to move, cartilage releases that synovial fluid back into the joint to reduce friction. Cartilage filled with fluid is eight times more slippery than ice.

Noisy Joints

Not all of the sounds in joints reflect damage to cartilage, but noises can be a sign that something is not quite right. In some individuals, ligaments make cracking and popping sounds as they pass over the joints or slide past bone. If a loose piece of bone or cartilage gets caught between the bone surfaces of a joint, any movement that frees the locked joint may result in a popping sound. Grinding noises can come from joints containing bones that have been roughened by the wearing away of large amounts of cartilage.

Sometimes people pop or crack some of their joints, especially the knuckles, on purpose. This can be done only with joints that hold synovial fluid, which in turn contains dissolved oxygen as well as carbon dioxide and nitrogen gases. Like the gases dissolved in any liquid, gases in synovial fluid are affected by pressure. The higher the pressure on a liquid, the more dissolved gases it can hold. That is why a sealed soda bottle loses some of its dissolved carbon dioxide when the cap is removed. Likewise, force on a joint stretches the capsule, increasing the volume of the capsule and simultaneously decreasing the pressure on the fluid within it. When pressure drops, some of the gases in the snyovial fluid come out of the solution. The popping sound is caused by the gases rapidly leaving the joint. The joint cannot be cracked again until gases have had time to dissolve in the fluid once more. This explains why a knuckle that was just cracked cannot be cracked again for another fifteen minutes or so.

One-Way Motion at Uniaxial Joints

The synovial joints of the body can produce different types and ranges of motion. These motions are dependent on the shapes of the bones that meet in the joint and the position of the ligaments. Some synovial joints permit only one type of movement, while others allow multiple movements. The different types of synovial joints are classified, based on the range of movement, as uniaxial, biaxial, or multiaxial joints.

The simplest synovial joints, uniaxial, permit movement in one direction only. Hinge joints, gliding joints, and pivot joints are examples of uniaxial joints. Hinge joints are found in the elbows, fingers, and toes. In a hinge joint, the rounded end of one bone fits into the concave indention on the other bone to form a hinge-shaped unit, similar to a hinge on a door. This type of joint allows bones to be moved back and forth but not rotated. Back-and-forth motion is called flexion and extension. In flexion, the joint bends, decreasing the angle between two bones. For example, a weight lifter bending an elbow and pulling a weight upward in a biceps curl performs a flexion. In extension, the opposite of flexion, the movement increases the angle between two bones by straightening a limb. A weight lifter working the arm's triceps muscle is performing an extension. This movement begins with weights in hands, elbows bent and close to the sides of the body, and the body bent forward slightly at the waist. The elbows are slowly unbent, and the weights pushed down and toward the back.

A gliding joint, another uniaxial type, allows two bones to move smoothly past each other. One of the articulating bones in a gliding joint is generally somewhat curved, while the other is flat. These types of joints are found between the carpal bones of the wrists and the tarsal bones of the ankles. Like hinge joints, gliding joints do not allow rotation and, compared to some types of synovial joints, permit only very limited mobility.

The pivot joint allows bones to turn or rotate around each other in one axis. There is a pivot joint between the first two vertebrae of the neck. Shaking the head from side to side is a result of motion at this pivot joint where the first cervical vertebra of the neck rotates on the second cervical vertebra. This motion is actually only a partial rotation, since the joint does not allow the head to spin completely

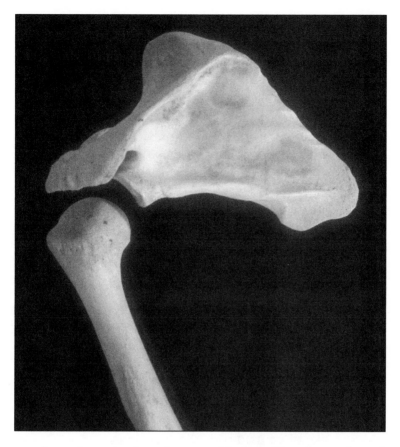

The shoulder's ball-and-socket joint allows for great range of motion but is also susceptible to injury.

on the axis, a motion that would sever blood vessels and nerves. Another pivot joint is found where the radius rotates over the ulna in the lower arm.

Two-Way Traffic Ahead

Bones that lie perpendicular to each other also need joints; otherwise, motion would be impossible. Two types of biaxial joints, the saddle and the condyloid, permit back-and-forth as well as side-to-side motion. Saddle joints received their name because the bones in them look like two miniature saddles that fit together. There are only two saddle joints in the human body, one in each thumb at the point where the thumb connects to the carpal, or hand, bone. With this important feature, called the opposable thumb, humans are able to use their hands to pick up, hold, and manipulate things. The saddle joints allow the thumbs to reach over and touch the tops of the fingers of that same hand. Without the saddle joints, simple tasks such as holding a glass of water or picking up a paper clip off a table would be virtually impossible.

The other biaxial joint, the condyloid, also moves from side to side and back and forth. Condyloids work much like saddle joints but have a different shape. They occur where a rounded oval part of a bone fits into a larger, egg-shaped socket, such as the joint formed where the radius fits into the carpal bone of the wrist. This joint affords the wrist a lot of flexibility.

The multiaxial joints of the human body can move in three ways: back and forth, side to side, and around. The largest multiaxial joints are the ball-and-socket type. In the ball-and-socket joint, the head of one bone fits into a concave depression in the other bone. The shoulders and hips are examples of ball-and-socket joints. Even though ball-and-socket joints have the advantage of a great range of motion, they are relatively unstable and thus susceptible to injury. The shoulder joint, the most mobile joint of the human body, is easily injured by the stress of repetitive motions like those used by baseball pitchers.

Making Joints Connect

Joints make possible a wide variety of motions. Along with the muscles and bones, each part of a joint plays an important role in completing a smooth motion. At the same time, joints prevent damage to the bones and muscles by bathing bone junctions in lubricating fluid and providing smooth cartilage surfaces for bones to slide across.

A common action like bending a knee may seem fairly simple. However, a closer look shows that when the knee bends to take a step, several things happen. The hamstring muscles, located in the back of the thigh, contract, bending the knee and pulling the leg up. At the same time, the quadriceps muscles, on the front of the thigh, relax to permit bending to occur. In the knee joint, cartilage and syno-vial fluid lubricate bones of both the thigh and leg to pre-vent them from rubbing against each other, and fluid-filled bursae provide extra cushioning. Five sturdy, supple liga-ments around the knee joint keep the bones connected to each other and in their proper places. Tendons attach the muscles of the thigh to the femur and those of the leg to the tibia and fibula. They also hold the kneecap in a protective position in front of the knee joint.

The joints of the human body are susceptible to injury, and they also undergo natural changes as a person ages. To maintain joint health, physicians recommend that adults

The radius and ulna bones (left) join together here with the humerus to form the elbow.

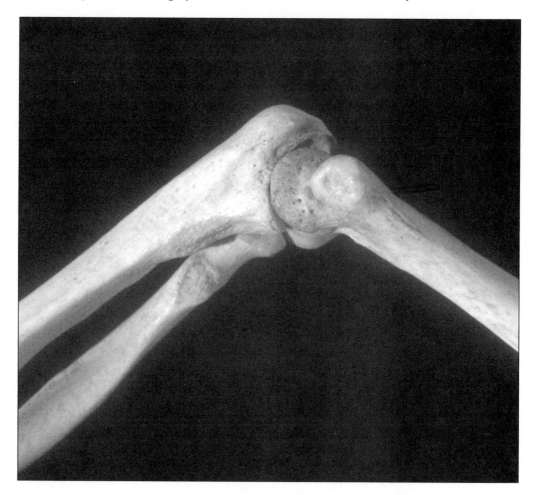

develop an exercise routine of moderate aerobic exercise, such as walking at least three or four times a week, combined with gentle stretching. Exercise should be started and stopped gradually, allowing muscles time to warm up and cool off. Stretching combined with exercise helps people maintain a healthy range of motion as they age.

Diseases and Disorders of the Musculo-skeletal System

4

Bone provides a record of the past, and much of the medical history of primitive man can be read in skeletal remains. Compared to other body parts, bones do not decay rapidly, so they supply information about many aspects of the lifestyles of ancient peoples. Bones also furnish scientists with information about prehistoric medical practices. For example, old skeletons show that breaks or fractures in the bones of early people often healed in proper alignment, suggesting that treatments such as simple splints and rest were used. Bones also tell researchers that primitive man performed crude amputations of limbs and fingers, most likely in an effort to save the lives of individuals with serious injuries. Another early surgical technique preserved in bone evidence is trephining of the skull, the carving of holes into the head of a living patient, perhaps to release evil spirits.

In more recent history, famous scientists and physicians have left written records about their studies of bone and muscle. Hippocrates (460–370 B.C.), celebrated as the father of medicine, described how he treated bones that had slipped out of their proper place in the joint. Aristotle (384–322 B.C.), a Greek teacher, analyzed the movements of animals and wrote descriptions of the mechanics of walking. Galen (A.D. 131–201), a Roman surgeon who served as the doctor for gladiators, is often considered the first practitioner of sports medicine. By tending the wounds of fighting men, he gained experience in treating injured muscle and bone. In his classic book, *On the Movements of Muscles*,

Galen described the mechanisms of movement, laying the foundation for the study of muscles. Galen was the first to propose two concepts that are well known today: that muscles' actions are controlled by some sort of signal from the brain and that muscles contract by shortening.

Galen's work stood unchallenged for centuries. During his lifetime, however, examination of cadavers (dead bodies)

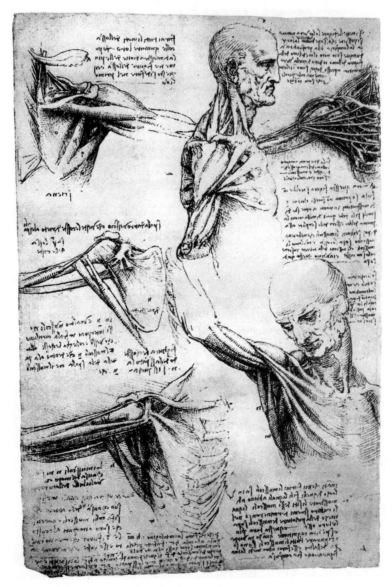

Leonardo da Vinci's remarkably accurate drawings helped to reveal faults in Galen's previous study of muscles.

was strictly forbidden. Consequently, he studied animals and drew parallels between them and humans. Over a thousand years later, Leonardo da Vinci (1452–1519), a skilled artist and engineer, was able to use cadavers to research a series of very accurate drawings of body structures. His pictures of bones, joints, and muscles showed details such as ball and socket joints and muscle insertions. Da Vinci's research revealed and corrected errors in Galen's work.

Today, physicians treat hundreds of different diseases and injuries of the musculoskeletal system. Modern man suffers from some of the same problems that plagued early humans. Bones still break, usually as the result of an accidental injury, and must be treated.

Breaking Up

Of all the body systems, the musculoskeletal is most prone to injury. Bones, muscles, and all of their supporting structures are intimately involved in the motions of everyday life. Athletes suffer more bone and muscle injuries than nonathletes because they push their body systems to perform at their physical limits. Knowledge gained in sports medicine, a field developed specifically to support athletes, can be applied to many musculoskeletal injuries that are similar to sports injuries but have different causes. Bone and muscle injuries range from mild and slightly uncomfortable to severe and extremely painful. Treatment depends on the specific injury but often includes rest, warm and cold compresses, elevation of the damaged area, and immobilization with splints or bandages.

Bones break because they are fairly rigid. When an outside force is applied to a bone, the bone gives a little as it absorbs much of the force. Children's bones are more flexible than those of adults, and they will bend as far as forty-five degrees. If a force is greater than a bone's ability to absorb it, however, the bone will break, just like a stick of wood snaps if it is bent too far. If the force applied is just a little more than the bone can support, then it may crack instead of break. Extreme forces, like those seen in car accidents and in falls from high places, may shatter bones into fragments.

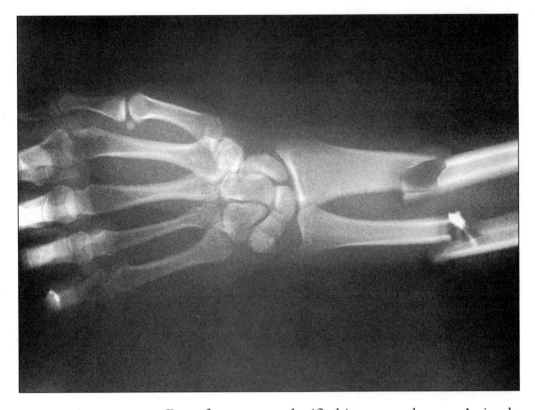

An X ray shows what is called a "simple," yet painful, fracture of the radius (top) and ulna (bottom) bones.

Bone fractures are classified into several types. A simple fracture is one in which the broken ends of the bone remain under the skin. If the bone is only cracked or bent, the damage is a greenstick fracture. A compression fracture results when a force presses one bone against another. If the vertebrae in the spinal column deteriorate, they can rub against one another and cause compression fractures. If the break causes fragments of bone to stick out through the skin, it is described as a compound fracture. Such a wound can be very serious, since piercing the skin exposes the bone and other internal structures to infectious agents. If several bone fragments are produced by an injuring force, the wound is described as a comminuted fracture. This type is often slow to heal because the blood supply to bone cells may have been compromised.

Any type of fracture can cause pain, swelling, limited motion, and inability to bear weight on the injured body part. Fractures are usually treated by immobilizing them in a cast or splint so that the natural healing abilities of the body can repair the damaged tissues.

Muscles, Tendons, and Ligaments Under Stress

Muscles can be damaged by misuse or overuse. Every time a muscle is repetitively exercised for long periods of time, some of its fibers are damaged or weakened. Such heavy muscle service also consumes all the glycogen stores in a muscle. It takes at least two days for the body to restore glycogen in muscle tissues and to heal damaged fibers. Therefore, heavy muscle work that occurs day after day does not give the muscles time to recuperate and increases the chance of injury.

Tendons and ligaments tear when they are required to bear more force than they can support. Joints are more likely to be injured if the tendons and ligaments in them are stretched past their normal limits. Improper stretching before movement or lack of adequate hydration can lead to stiffness in tendons, increasing the chance that they will tear or stretch. Once damaged, a tendon often swells, causing an uncomfortable or painful condition called tendonitis. The Achilles tendon, which connects the calf muscles to the heel, can develop tendonitis from an injury or from overuse. The Achilles tendon is essential in movements such as walking, running, and jumping. Tendons that bend the wrist forward and back are also subject to damage. A condition known as tennis elbow sends pain along the forearm when the wrist tendons are bent.

Another common ailment associated with tendons is carpal tunnel syndrome, which can cause a burning pain in the hand and fingers, numbness or tingling in the fingers, and weakness in the hands that makes simple manual tasks difficult or uncomfortable. The condition gets its name from a passageway in the wrist, the carpal tunnel, that holds a nerve traveling from the forearm to the hand. The tunnel is made of bone on the bottom and sides and of tendon on the top. Like all tendons, the carpal tunnel tendon is covered with a lubricating membrane, the synovium, which can swell after long hours of repeated motions at the computer or from bending, pushing, or pulling. Swelling may compress the nerve against the tendon, causing uncomfortable symptoms.

Further up the arm, the tendons that hold the upper arm in the shoulder joint form an area known as the rotator cuff. Tendonitis of the rotator cuff can be caused by swimming, pitching a baseball, or serving a tennis ball, as well as any other motion that moves the arm over the head repeatedly. When the arm moves over the head, the top of the ulna rubs against part of the shoulder joint, damaging the tendons and ligaments and causing pain. In severe cases, the tendons actually tear away from the bone.

The knee is another active joint that is frequently damaged. Articular cartilage tears occur in people who stress their knees in sports or at work. A section of the cartilage in the knee, the portion referred to as the meniscus, is especially vulnerable to injury. A meniscus runs down the outside edge of each knee joint and crosses the joint between the two joined bones. Most menisci have no blood supply, so once they are injured, it is difficult for them to heal. As a person ages, their menisci deteriorate, and the likelihood of knee injury increases.

Bad to the Bone

Since bone provides the body's framework as well as part of the structure that allows movement, diseases of the bone can be deforming and debilitating. For bones to form normally, adequate supplies of calcium and phosphorus must be present in the diet. Bone formation also requires vitamin D, which can be supplied by the diet or manufactured by the body when it is exposed to sunlight. Vitamin D is essential for absorption and use of calcium and phosphorus in bones. Children who do not get adequate supplies of minerals, or who are not exposed to enough sunlight, may develop rickets, a disease in which bones do not harden, sometimes

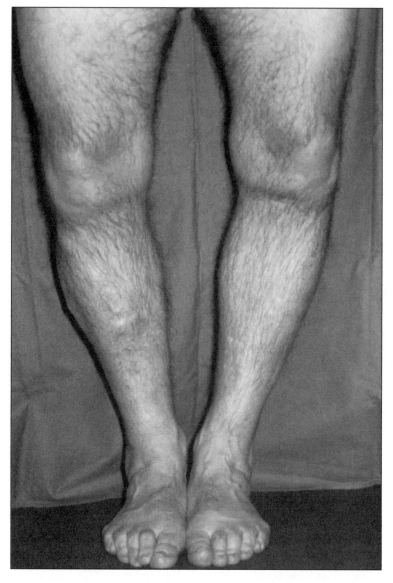

This man's bowed legs are the results of rickets, a deformity caused by a vitamin D deficiency.

resulting in skeletal deformities. The bones of children with rickets are soft and tend to bend, so some develop bowed or knock-kneed legs because their bones cannot support the weight of their bodies. Other symptoms include a curved spine, a sternum that protrudes forward, and nodules on the ends of ribs. In severe cases, lack of calcium, which plays an essential role in muscle contraction, causes muscles to be flabby. Severely affected children have square, large heads, delayed appearance of teeth, and a potbelly. Many of these symptoms can be reduced with supplements of vitamin D, calcium, phosphorus, and exposure to light.

Unlike rickets, which occurs most often in children, another bone disease, osteoporosis, is more commonly seen in middle-aged and elderly women. Although the disease can affect both sexes, women are especially vulnerable because their bodies stop making estrogen, a female hormone, after midlife. Estrogen helps form bone.

Osteoporosis causes bone to become thin and weak and therefore easy to break. Normally, bone density increases each year up until age thirty, at which time it begins to slowly decrease. The body has built-in mechanisms for maintaining adequately strong bones through all stages of life, but changes in nutrition, exercise, exposure to sunlight, and levels of hormones can disturb those mechanisms.

Although some people with osteoporosis develop few symptoms, others lose so much of their supporting bone structure that bones cave in or break. Broken vertebrae cause a round-backed posture called dowager's hump that is sometimes seen in women. The chronic back pain that can result from these breaks may severely limit movement. Generally, the pain in the back starts suddenly and worsens when standing or sitting. Other bones can fracture, or break easily from minor injury. The elderly are particularly at risk of breaking the hipbones during a fall. In older people with osteoporosis, breaks heal slowly. The axiom "An ounce of prevention is worth a pound of cure" is very true in the case of osteoporosis. Prevention involves good nutrition and weight-bearing exercise to maintain strong bone structure.

Another malady that appears more often in people over forty years old than in younger people is Paget's disease, which causes areas of the skeleton to enlarge and soften. Although any bone can be affected, those most often involved are the pelvis, femur, skull, vertebrae, clavicle, and humerus. Normally, two types of bone cells, osteoclasts and osteoblasts, continually rebuild the skeleton. Osteoclasts break down old bone and osteoblasts build new bone in a rhythm that maintains a strong, healthy skeleton. In Paget's disease, both types of cells become overactive, destroying and depositing bone at such rapid rates that the resulting bone is oversized but weak.

The cause of this abnormal bone cell activity is not known, although researchers suspect that a virus is to blame. People who suffer Paget's disease display a variety of symptoms, depending on which bones are affected. If the skull is involved, the forehead may become heavy and thick. Enlarged bones of the skull can compress areas of the inner ear, causing hearing loss, or parts of the brain, producing headaches. When bones of the spine are involved, they can collapse on nerves in the vertebrae, pinching them and causing pain or paralysis in the limbs. Hipbones and

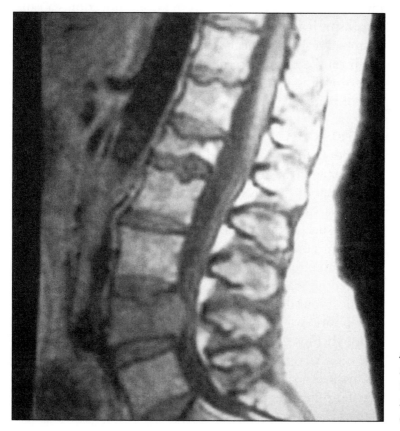

A spinal cross section shows deformed and thickened vertebrae, symptoms of Paget's disease.

leg bones can become deformed, resulting in difficulty standing or walking.

Bones, like other tissues throughout the body, can become infected by disease-causing agents, especially bacteria and fungi. Osteomyelitis is an inflammation of a bone, usually due to infectious agents that have reached the bone from the bloodstream, through an open wound, or from infections in neighboring soft tissues. Infection-causing organisms that travel in blood may enter the body any time a foreign material, such as a hypodermic needle, is introduced. Therefore, people who undergo regular medical treatment that involves needles, as well as those who inject illegal drugs, are at higher risk of infection than others. Infectious agents can also enter the bone directly if the bone breaks and sticks out of the skin or during surgery that involves placing screws or bolts in bones. Infection-causing organisms living in soft tissue can also transfer to bone. For example, a slow-to-heal skin ulcer or an infected gum or tooth can be the source of infection in bones of the skull. Osteomyelitis results in swelling and pain in the affected area of bone.

In the Joint

Like bone, joints may develop conditions that result from the wear and tear of normal aging, from injury, from inherited conditions, or from illness. The joints that are affected the most are usually the ones that support the body's weight, such as the lower spine, hips, and knees. Joint diseases can cause pain and interfere with normal movements and flexibility.

Force can damage a joint or the tendons, ligaments, and muscles around it. A force can dislocate a bone from its normal position in a joint. Any bone can be dislocated, although those in the shoulders and fingers are the most common victims. For healing to occur, the bone must be put back in its correct place, then immobilized while tendons and ligaments heal. A sprain results when a joint is turned in such a way that the ligaments are damaged. Some sprained areas swell and discolor because tissues and blood vessels surrounding the joint are also injured. The type of neck injury called a whiplash is a sprain of the vertebrae of the neck. If the damaging force tears muscles or tendons around a joint, the injury is called a strain or a pulled muscle. Strains can result from excessive exercise or from suddenly using a muscle that is not warmed up.

The most common disorder of joints is osteoarthritis, a disease that affects the cartilage lining the inside of joints. Joints are designed so that the bones within them can glide effortlessly across each other on a layer of slick cartilage. In osteoarthritis, that lubricating layer of cartilage thins or wears away. Destruction of cartilage causes the development of tiny pits in the underlying bone. Eventually the bones are not able to move smoothly, and other parts of the joint, such as the synovial capsule, ligaments, and tendons, are also damaged.

By age forty, most people have some osteoarthritis, although few display symptoms. When symptoms do appear, they come gradually, usually in one joint at a time. Joints of the fingers, neck, back, toes, hips, and knees are usually affected first. Pain may be most intense after a period of exercise. In the mornings, those areas may feel stiff but often limber up with movement. In serious conditions, joints may continue to lose their flexibility until they become fixed in a bent position, and bony growths may appear at the ends of fingers. Even though joints are stiff, the best treatment is a combination of stretching and strengthening exercises.

Internal Conflict

Rheumatoid arthritis is a more damaging and crippling disease than osteoarthritis, and it results from an entirely different process. In rheumatoid arthritis, the body's immune system attacks the cartilage in its own joints, inflaming the synovial membranes that line them. The inflammation, in turn, causes a joint to be stiff and makes movement painful. Eventually cartilage, ligaments, tendons, and bone within the affected joints show deterioration, and the bones grate when they move against one another. Symptoms may appear suddenly, and they usually affect the body in a uniform pattern; if one hand begins to hurt, so does the other hand.

The first joints to be affected are often the small ones like fingers, toes, and wrists. Continued loss of cartilage at the ends of the bones causes the formation of a certain type of scar tissue, which can be converted into bone, fusing the ends of the bones in a joint. Over time, such fusion immobilizes and stiffens a joint, causing it to increase in size and become misshapen. The hand joints of rheumatoid arthritis patients often fuse, causing the fingers to turn to the side. In some cases, hard knots form under the skin near diseased joints. In rheumatoid arthritis, the immune system may also damage other areas of the body such as the lungs, blood vessels, and lymph nodes. Unlike osteoarthritis, joints in rheumatoid arthritis need more rest than exercise to avoid swelling.

Extremely crooked fingers and misshapen joints are a sure sign of rheumatoid arthritis.

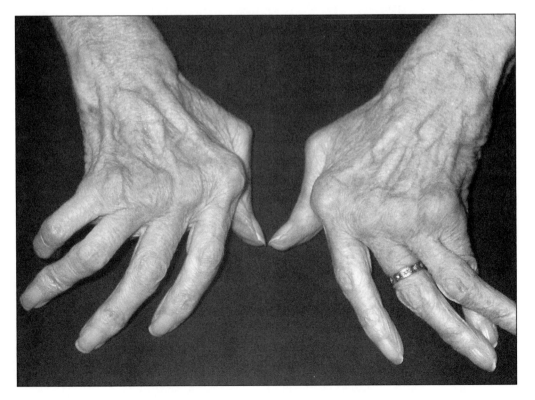

Inflammation and pain can also be caused by gout, a disease in which uric acid crystals are deposited in joints. Uric acid is generated by the normal breakdown of genetic material in worn-out cells, so it is present in the blood at all times. However, if levels of the acid become high due to disease, some of it crystallizes in the joints. The body's immune system treats these crystals as foreign invaders and attacks them, causing pain and swelling. Gout causes severe pain in one or two joints. The joints swell, and the skin over them becomes red. Joints in the big toe, instep, ankle, knee, and wrist are most often affected. These areas may be susceptible because they are located on the extremities, and crystals form in places that are cooler than the core of the body. People who are susceptible to gout are encouraged to follow two strategies: drink large quantities of water to flush the body of uric acid and eat foods that generate uric acid, such as those that are high in protein, in small quantities.

Muscles on Strike

Muscles are tissues that work with bones to produce movement. Like bones and joints, they can be injured or infected. One group of wasting muscle diseases is collectively known as the muscular dystrophies. The most common form in children, Duchenne's muscular dystrophy, is caused by a malfunctioning gene on the X chromosome, one of the two sex chromosomes. Females have two X chromosomes, and boys have one X and one Y chromosome. If a girl has a flaw on one of her X chromosomes, the other chromosome compensates for it by operating correctly. However, since males have only one X chromosome, they develop the disease if they inherit the one faulty gene. That is why boys are much more likely to suffer Duchenne's than girls. The imperfect gene does not produce a muscle protein needed to maintain the structure of muscle cells.

Between the ages of three and seven, symptoms of Duchenne's muscular dystrophy begin appearing. One of the first is a weakness in the lower body that makes it difficult to walk, climb stairs, or rise from a seated position.

Eventually, symptoms worsen as the condition spreads to other muscles throughout the body. Affected muscles become larger than normal, but they are extremely weak. Many times the heart muscles are damaged, too. Muscles around joints contract, bending the spine, elbows, and knees. A wheelchair is usually needed by age twelve. Young people with Duchenne's are in a weakened physical condition, so they are highly susceptible to infectious diseases; consequently, most die in their teens. No treatment can cure the disease, but physical therapy that stretches and exercises joints can help relax them, providing some degree of comfort.

Myotonic dystrophy is the most common form of adult muscular dystrophy. People with this disease suffer from constant muscle contraction. Prolonged contractions make muscles weak, and, as a consequence, they waste away. Like Duchenne's, myotonic dystrophy is caused by a malfunctioning gene. However, the gene involved is located on one of the body chromosomes, not on a sex chromosome, so males and females are affected equally. This gene is dominant, so its presence will mask a functional, recessive gene. The faulty gene can cause other health problems including loss of muscle tone, irregular heartbeats, diabetes, and mental retardation.

Like bones and joints, muscles can be damaged by diseases of the immune system. Myasthenia gravis, whose name originates from Latin and Greek words that mean "serious muscle weakness," causes weakness of skeletal muscles. The disease appears between the ages of twenty and forty and is more common in women than men. Weakness is most pronounced after periods of activity, and it improves after rest. Typically, muscles of the face, jaw, and mouth are affected. In fact, the first symptom is often a weakness of the muscles in the eyelids, which causes drooping. As the disease progresses, it interferes with normal speech and swallowing. Myasthenia gravis is due to the interruption of the electrical impulse that travels from the brain to a muscle. At the muscle end of a nerve fiber, thou-

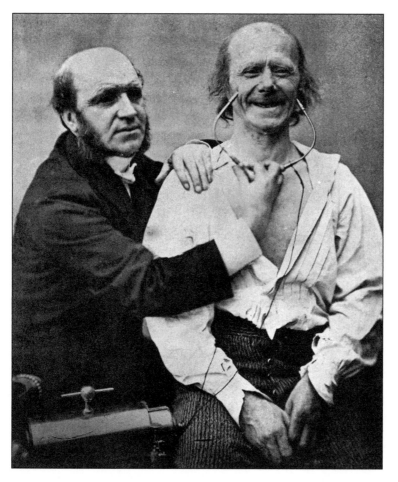

French physician Duchenne uses an electronic device to stimulate his patient's facial muscles.

sands of tiny sacs hold neurotransmitters that are designed to carry an electrical signal across the gap between a nerve cell and a muscle cell. Special receptors on the muscle cell act as docks that receive the neurotransmitters. Docking is essential for the electrical impulse to stimulate a muscle cell. In myasthenia gravis, antibodies, which are chemicals made by the body's own immune system, block the receptors, preventing muscle cell activation.

It is a Wrap

To bring attention to the prevalence of musculoskeletal disorders, the World Health Organization (WHO), headquartered in Geneva, Switzerland, designated the years

2002 through 2011 as the Bone and Joint Decade. During this time, WHO hopes to increase public awareness of muscle and bone disorders and raise money to fund research in this field to facilitate the advancement of treatments. Currently, musculoskeletal problems touch the lives of millions of people worldwide. The number of those affected will double by 2020 as the world's population ages.

In the United States, almost every adult injures his or her back at least once, and one out of seven Americans suffer from chronic muscle or bone problems. Injuries and diseases related to the musculosketal system are the primary cause of disability in working-age people. From 1992 to 1994, injuries to bone and muscle accounted for two-thirds of all injuries reported to medical practitioners.

Arthritis is the leading chronic disease of the elderly and a more frequent cause of limitation than heart disease, diabetes, or cancer. This is certainly an area where research is warranted.

Advances in Musculoskeletal Medical Technology

5

As long as humans have been on Earth, they have sustained injuries. Consequently, medicine men, bonesetters, shamans, and other early practitioners have treated damage to muscles and bones for thousands of years. However, today's treatments for diseases that afflict the musculoskeletal system are relatively young. Much of the foundational work was done by great scientists in the last three hundred years.

At the age of eighty-one, Nicholas Andry (1658–1759), a professor of medicine in Paris, published *Orthopaedia: The Art of Correcting and Preventing Deformities in Children.* Andry was the first to use the word *orthopaedics*, a term derived from the Greek words for "straight" and "child," to describe a branch of medicine. He taught that parents could use the strategies outlined in his book to help prevent skeletal deformities in children. Some honor him as the father of orthopedics, but critics feel that his primary contribution to science was the now famous term *orthopedics* rather than medical research. In modern medicine, orthopedics refers to the branch of medicine that treats diseases, injuries, and conditions of the musculoskeletal system.

John Hunter (1728–1793) was a military surgeon serving British troops in the Seven Years War. He later established a research center in London where he taught medicine. Although he had little formal training, Hunter used a scientific approach to problem solving that paved the way for

A sixteenth-century drawing demonstrates an early orthopedic treatment for a dislocated knee.

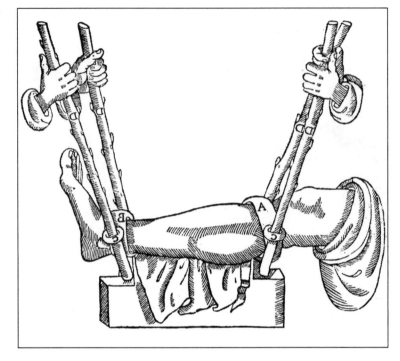

many later developments in orthopedics. He was one of the first physicians to document the need to immobilize an injured bone or joint until it had healed. Unlike most other physicians of his day, who were quick to propose amputation and other extreme therapeutic measures, Hunter taught that the body is capable of healing itself; the surgeon's job is to help the natural process along.

Today, a physician follows a standard set of procedures when seeking the cause of a musculoskeletal problem. Each step in the procedure provides new clues, filling in the blank spaces of the puzzling ailment. The first step is usually a medical history, which gives a physician insight into a patient's general health as well as the health of that patient's family. A physical examination is an external inspection of a patient's body to see if more evidence can be gathered. To supplement this preliminary information, medical tests may be needed. Blood and urine can be analyzed for abnormalities. Imaging techniques such as X rays, CT scans, and MRI scans are invaluable for their ability to take pictures of the inside of the body. Sometimes a physician will also need to examine a sample of bone or muscle, in which case a small piece of suspicious tissue is removed for closer examination under a microscope. Armed with information from all these sources, a physician may recommend an appropriate treatment.

Sticks and Stones Can Break My Bones

In treating bone fractures, physicians today follow the same basic procedures used by early doctors such as John Hunter: realign the broken bone, immobilize it, and give it time to grow back together. In any fracture, the first step is to reduce, or put back together, the individual pieces of bone. Bones that are not properly realigned are likely to mend in the wrong position, causing structural problems.

Though it may look like a medieval torture device, this apparatus actually sets and repositions fractured bones.

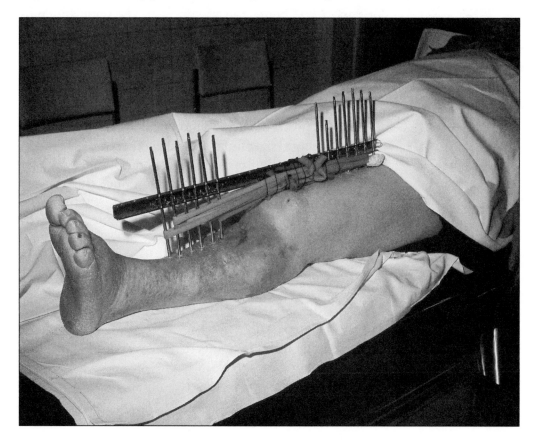

Generally, broken bones in a closed fracture can be gently manipulated back in place by a trained medical practitioner. If bone is shattered into several pieces, it may be necessary to perform an open reduction: a surgical procedure during which the bone pieces are repositioned, then held in place with metal screws, plates, or rods inserted into the center of the bones. Once all misplaced bones are correctly positioned, the damaged area is immobilized so that the body can heal the broken bones.

A cast is an inflexible plaster or fiberglass shell that stabilizes broken bones until they have healed. A broken arm encased in a cast will remain immobilized, facilitating healing, until the cast is removed. Broken bones can also be immobilized by external fixation, a method of inserting pins or screws through the skin and muscle and into the bone above and below the fracture site. The stabilizing pins or screws are then connected to a metal bar outside skin. The bar holds bones in proper position and is removed once the injury has healed.

Some forms of energy stimulate bone growth. Magnetism and electrical energy have been used for some time to mend bone after a fracture or to speed incorporation of bone used in a graft. Recent research indicates that another form of energy, sound waves, has a similar effect. Fresh bone injuries heal faster when treated with low-intensity ultrasound energy than injuries that are not exposed to any source of energy. Such treatments are easy and painless. A small, battery-operated device placed on the area over the break generates ultrasound energy at the injury site. A once-a-day, twenty-minute treatment is all that is needed to accelerate healing.

The Knee Bone's Connected to the Leg Bone

Knees and hips are large joints that are responsible for supporting much of the body's weight. As a result, they are vulnerable to wear and tear and to injury. Several surgical procedures have been developed to repair or replace these joints when they are severely damaged.

Knee pain can result from a torn meniscus or damaged knee ligament. If a piece of meniscal tissue gets caught between the bones of the knee joint, the femur and tibia, pain and swelling can result. A damaged meniscus can be removed or repaired, and torn knee ligaments can be reconstructed. All of these procedures can be accomplished by arthroscopy, a surgical technique that requires only small incisions and uses miniaturized surgical instruments.

During arthroscopy, a thin tube, or catheter, is inserted into a joint through a small incision. Once in place, an arthroscope, a fiberoptic telescope about the diameter of a pencil, is inserted through the catheter. When the scope is correctly positioned, fluid is pumped into the joint to distend it and allow the physician to see the internal structures. One or more additional catheters also supply entry for the working ends of surgical instruments as small as one-tenth of an inch. Inside the knee, tissues can be probed and examined, and surgery can be performed. Because incisions are small, this type of surgery is usually done on an outpatient basis, and the patient can walk on crutches within forty-eight hours. After the knee heals, patients must participate in a rehabilitation program to strengthen the muscles around the knee.

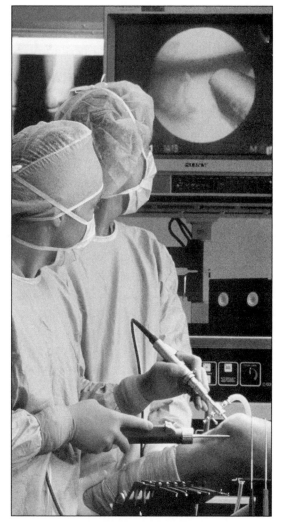

Surgeons perform arthroscopic knee surgery in which tissues can be examined and treated with relatively little trauma.

Both knee and hip joints can be severely damaged by osteoarthritis. Loss of cartilage at these joints causes pain, which can severely restrict movement and interfere with a person's day-to-day life. Even the ankle, foot, shoulder, elbow, and finger joints can be targets of osteoarthritic damage. Any of these joints can be operated on to relieve pain and restore freedom of movement.

In a surgical procedure, the arthritic or damaged joint is completely removed and replaced with an artificial joint called a prosthesis. The hip, a large ball-and-socket joint, is one of the most common targets of joint replacement. The upper end of the femur creates the ball in this joint, and part of the pelvis forms the socket. During surgery, long incisions in the thigh permit the surgeon to move aside muscle and other surrounding tissues to get to the joint. The damaged head of the femur is sawed off, and a metal ball is cemented to the bone. Metals commonly used are strong ones such as stainless steel, titanium, and alloys of cobalt and chromium. The damaged part of the hip socket is also removed, and a durable plastic socket is implanted in its place. Once all the new parts are securely in position, the incision is closed. Typically, a patient spends three to five days in the hospital. The day after surgery, the patient is asked to walk slowly, an experience that can be painful because the muscles around the joint are weakened after the trauma of surgery. However, patients heal completely over the next few weeks. Ongoing exercise is a very important part of recovery. Currently, a total joint replacement lasts about ten years, but orthopedic surgeons are working with engineers to find materials that will last longer.

The newest approach to hip surgery is to use smaller incisions and arthroscopic techniques to repair the damaged joint. Arthroscopic hip replacement surgery can be accomplished with two one-and-a-half-inch incisions, whereas the traditional surgery needed a twelve-inch incision in the thigh. Surgeons push the components of the new hip through these tiny openings and assemble them inside the body. This technique avoids cutting the large muscles of the leg, which take a long time to heal. Arthroscopic hip surgery can be done on an outpatient basis, and the patient can go home the same day with little pain.

Balloon in the Backbone

Bones in the spine that are weakened and fractured due to osteoarthritis can also be surgically repaired. At the University of California in San Francisco, orthopedic surgeons are studying a new technique called kyphoplasty. This procedure helps restore normal shape and function to vertebrae that have caved in. In this procedure, a small incision is made on each side of a damaged vertebra, and tiny, hollow tubes are inserted through the incision. Another thinner tube, tipped with an inflatable balloon, is introduced through the first tube. Once the balloon is positioned inside the vertebra, it is inflated, lifting the shattered pieces of bone. After the bone fragments have been moved back to their original positions, a cementlike material is injected into the space to fix the vertebral parts in place. This technique is a big improvement over an older procedure in which cement was injected into a collapsed vertebra with no attempt to correct its shape. Kyphoplasty results in improvement in spine function and much less pain.

Revitalized Vitamin

Some bone damage is not the result of damage or injury but of conditions that cause loss of bone or inability of bone to form properly. Vitamin D is a nutrient that is known to play a vital role in bone formation, so people who are at risk for weak bones are often given supplements of vitamin D. Supplements seem to promote small increases in bone mass, but sometimes these modest gains are not enough to be helpful. Researchers have recently developed a new, more promising form of vitamin D that has a dramatic impact on bone mass. Lead by Hector F. DeLuca at the University of Wisconsin-Madison, preliminary experiments suggest that the newest form of vitamin D, known as 2MD, aggressively stimulates bone growth. In the lab, it has been used to grow bone cells in flasks and to promote the growth of bone in experimental animals.

Postmenopausal women are the largest group of people who suffer from osteoporosis, or loss of bone mass. Older women lose bone when their bodies stop producing the female hormone, estrogen. To create a similar condition in lab rats, DeLuca's group removed the rats' ovaries, putting the female rats into an induced menopause and causing bone loss. To test the new supplement, the experimental animals were given the 2MD form of vitamin D. The investigators reported that the rats showed a 9 percent increase in total body bone mass, a much greater increase than has been previously seen with other forms of vitamin D. Scientists believe that this potent compound works by stimulating growth of osteoblasts.

A doctor explains osteoporosis, a condition that affects many postmenopausal women.

Borrowed Bone

In some conditions, researchers have found a way to help the body strengthen existing bone tissue. Bone-marrow transplants may be another tool in the doctor's bag for helping patients rebuild bone. In the past, bone-marrow transplants have been successful in treating several inherited diseases in other body systems, as well as some forms of blood cancer. When healthy cells from a donor's marrow are injected into a recipient, they assist the recipient's body in its fight against disease. Recently, bone-marrow transplants have been found to slow the progress of a relatively rare, but devastating, bone disease.

Children who suffer from the inherited disease osteogenesis imperfecta have very weak skeletons, so they are often deformed and extremely small. Because their bodies do not make all of the materials necessary to build strong bone, their bones are fragile and break easily. In some cases, children's skeletons are so weak that parents have accidentally broken bones while changing diapers. There is no cure for the condition and very few treatments. The traditional way of reinforcing these weak bones is a surgical procedure in which physicians insert rods into long bones, giving them more strength.

A study by Edwin M. Horwitz at St. Jude Children's Research Hospital in Memphis, Tennessee, is casting new light on this bleak picture. Working with a small group of very fragile children, Horwitz wanted to find out if his young patients could be helped by donations of bone cells from a sibling. Transplants of bone marrow from healthy children to their sick brothers or sisters yielded promising results: Horwitz found that bones in the sick children strengthened and grew. One of the children in the experimental group was a thirteen-month-old who had already suffered thirty-seven fractures. Six months after a transplant, this same child had suffered only three fractures and had gained bone mass.

Cells Under Construction

One of the newest technologies in treatment of bone diseases sounds like a story line from science fiction. Tissue engineering is a procedure that involves removing bone and cartilage cells from a patient's body, working with them in a lab, then replacing them. Back in the patient, these improved cells promote growth of bone and cartilage. This technique holds promise for people suffering from osteoarthritis and other conditions that damage joints. Currently, three types of tissue engineering are being explored.

One type of tissue treatment is called enzyme engineering. Enzymes are compounds made in the body that speed up chemical reactions. One cause of the loss of cartilage by osteoarthritis patients is the presence in their joints of an enzyme that stimulates the breakdown of cartilaginous tissue. Scientists are working on ways to alter, or genetically engineer, cells in the joint so that they will be able to destroy these enzymes, preventing further damage to cartilage. To do this, scientists must perfect a method of removing some of the cells from a joint, genetically changing them so that they produce chemicals that inhibit the destructive enzymes and then injecting the altered cells back into the joint.

Another approach in tissue engineering is cartilage cell replacement. Unlike other tissues in the body, cartilage does not heal itself if it is damaged. To compensate for this disadvantage, researchers are removing cartilage cells from patients' joints and using them to grow new populations of cartilage cells. In the lab, a donor's cartilage cells are placed in a flask with nutrients. Meanwhile, the patient goes about normal day-to-day activities. After a few days, the cells have divided so many times that the flask is covered with millions of the patient's own cartilage cells. These are then injected back into the patient's joint. A small piece of periosteum, the tissue that covers bone, is taken from another bone and then sewn over the site of injection to hold the cells in place. So far, this technique helps reduce the pain in joints, but scientists emphasize that it replaces cartilage rather than repairing it. However, they see the repair of damaged cells as their next challenge.

One avenue being pursued is to grow new cartilage cells from stem cells. Stem cells are simple, primitive cell forms that have the ability to change into other kinds of cells.

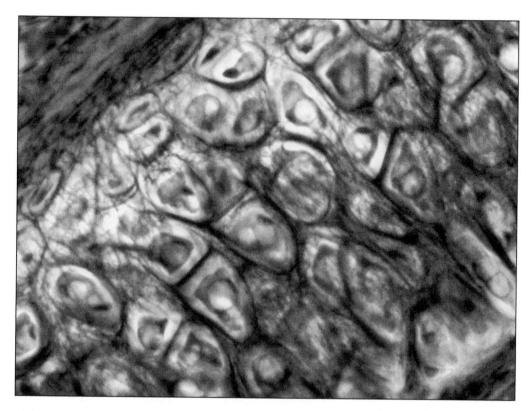

Consequently, stem cells can be the source of any type of tissue. Scientists hope that stem-cell research will lead to the development of a form of cartilage that can regenerate naturally and help heal a damaged joint. Such cells could also be used to regrow the cartilage in damaged parts of the ears, nose, and other cartilaginous structures. As a result, much reconstructive surgery could be avoided. This work is in its early stages at Johns Hopkins University, where researchers have stimulated the stem cells of adult goats to grow into cartilage-type tissue.

Cartilage cells like these offer great promise in new research on tissue engineering.

From Pegs to Processors

If large structures, such as a leg or a hand, are lost because of disease and injury, they can sometimes be replaced with artificial limbs called prostheses. The oldest known prosthetic legs are peg legs, wooden pegs that were strapped to an amputee's stump to help support the body weight. A peg leg is described as a static prosthesis because it does not employ the use of electronics. Newer artificial limbs, known as dynamic prostheses, take advantage of the electricity produced naturally by the body. When a person tenses muscles, those muscles produce a small electric current. Dynamic prostheses can detect that current and transmit signals to a device such as an artificial hand or foot.

Prosthetics can be custom-made for amputees to ensure a good fit. A person who has lost the lower leg, but not the knee, can have a socket created to fit over the remaining part of leg. The socket is molded from a cast of the leg. A protective sock is worn over the stump of the leg, between the leg and the socket. In the past, it has been difficult to create a socket that fits perfectly. However, the availability of new materials has made it possible to create better-fitting sockets. Silicone liners and gel-like padding make prostheses more comfortable and help hold them snugly in place.

In above-the-knee amputees, the knee joint is the trickiest and most important part of the prosthesis. In early versions, when an amputee lifted a leg to take a step, the lower portion of the prosthetic leg was designed to swing forward automatically at a set rate. The rate of swing and resistance of the knee joint had to be preset, and these two values determined the speed at which an amputee could walk. It was not easy to adjust the speed if the wearer wanted to change his or her pace. The advent of computer chips solved this problem. Microprocessors are capable of monitoring the position of the knee constantly. If the wearer starts walking faster, the computer detects the change and adjusts the resistance of the knee joint and the position of the lower leg to accommodate the new pace. In the newest artificial limbs, sensors can detect electrical stimulation from muscles in the user's leg. This permits the user to control the settings on the artificial leg through muscle contractions.

Functional prosthetic feet have been a challenge to create. The first prosthetic feet, which were stiff, were primarily designed to look like real feet. Today's version of a foot looks very different from the real thing but acts a lot like the genuine article. Made of a new material called carbon fiber, the newest prosthetic foot can absorb the shock of a step. When walking, the new foot pushes off from the ground and then springs back into shape, giving the user a little push just like a normal foot would. For walking, there is a so-called soft foot that gives only a little spring with each step. However, for running, stiffer feet are designed to give the wearer more push or bounce. These state-of-the-art artificial feet, which look something like bent spoons, can be

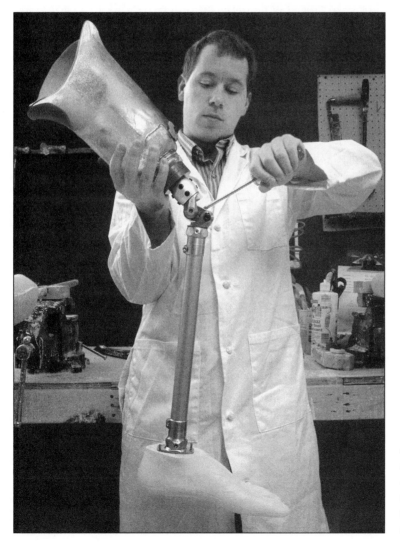

A designer carefully adjusts a prosthetic leg. Continuing advances improve the feel and function of prosthetics.

covered to look more like real feet and to allow the user to wear shoes.

Designers are working on a device called a Smart Lower Limb that will soon be available for amputees who have lost a foot or leg. This computer-enhanced prosthetic will be equipped with sensors that provide constant feedback to a computer about the position of the limb, stability, and balance. As all this information is fed into the microprocessor, the computer will tell the Smart Limb what to do next. These advances will enable amputees to walk in a more natural manner.

Skeleton Inside Out

Some of medicine's greatest advances have been closely tied to research conducted by the armed forces. Currently, the U.S. Defense Advanced Research Projects Agency is developing an exoskeleton suit to put on ground troops. Even though humans have a durable support system that provides them with great flexibility, an internal skeleton does not provide as much strength as an external one. An exoskeleton would let troops run faster, leap great heights, and carry heavy equipment. One therapeutic application for such a suit would be to provide strength and stability to people with muscle- or bone-wasting diseases.

A wearable exoskeleton would enhance many abilities. Early studies indicate that a wearer would be able to lift a 250-pound object as if it weighed a mere 10 pounds. People normally walk at a pace of four to six miles per hour, but a soldier carrying a 150-pound pack cannot sustain that speed over a long distance. However, with an exoskeleton, a fully loaded trooper could speed along at ten miles per hour.

The suit is far from completion because there are many challenges that must be solved. An exoskeleton must be made of a durable, lightweight, flexible material. It also needs to be easy to control so a wearer can carry out normal functions while using it. The skeleton must move smoothly, without the awkwardness of a machine so the wearer is quick and agile. Proponents believe, however, that these challenges are not insurmountable. Each generation of scientists builds on the knowledge of the previous generation. The discoveries that have been made and the problems that have been solved in the last twenty years would have sounded like science fantasy to our great-grandfathers. Exoskeletons are just one of the previously unimaginable breakthroughs hoped for in the twenty-first century.

Muscle and Bone

The two types of tissues that are responsible for movement are bone and muscle. Muscles apply force to bones by contracting. Each of the more than six hundred muscles is made up of long, thin cells containing thousands of microscopic strands of stretchy protein. All muscles are controlled by nerves that have direct links to the brain and spinal cord.

Bone is a living tissue just like muscle. Bone is constantly in a state of flux as cells dissolve old bone and deposit new. In this recycling activity, bone acts as a mineral bank that accepts deposits and makes withdrawals of calcium to keep this mineral's levels within the optimal range.

Research to find cures and treatments for musculoskeletal disorders is ongoing. Some of the newest research is being done during space travel. It is well known that weightlessness causes muscle wasting because, without gravity, muscles do not have a force to work against. That is one of the reasons astronauts feel weak and have trouble standing after a long flight. For now, this is a minor problem that corrects itself after a period of time back on Earth. However, in the future, it could be a more serious problem. In the future, astronauts who are already working in space stations for several months at a time will spend even longer periods at their posts. Plans are also being made to send astronauts on extended voyages in space. What is learned in space medicine will help provide treatments for people who suffer from bone- and muscle-wasting conditions.

GLOSSARY

articulate: To bring together at a joint.

cartilage: The slippery tissue within joints that enables bones to move against one another with little friction.

diaphysis: The shaft of a long bone, located between the epiphyses.

endoskeleton: The support structure within the body of an organism.

epiphyseal plate: An area of cartilage seen in young, growing bone.

epiphysis: The end of a long bone and the point at which two bones articulate.

exoskeleton: The support structure outside of the body of an organism.

fontanels: The soft areas of an infant's skull that are covered with fibrous membranes rather than bone.

fracture: A break in a bone.

glucose: The sugar used by cells to produce energy.

glycogen: A form of stored glucose.

haversian canals: The central canals running through the length of a bone that carry nerves and blood vessels.

insertion: The end of a muscle that is attached to a movable bone.

intervertebral disks: The areas of cartilage between vertebrae.

joint: The point at which two bones come together.

ligament: A strong, connective tissue that holds bones together at joints.

marrow: The soft tissue within the shaft of a bone.

motor neuron: A nerve that connects a muscle fiber to the spinal cord or brain.

neurotransmitters: The chemicals stored in vesicles of nerve cells that carry electrical impulses from a nerve to the target cell.

origin: The end of a muscle that is attached to an immovable bone.

ossification: The process of bone formation.

osteoblasts: Immature, bone-forming cells.

osteoclasts: Bone-dissolving cells.

osteocytes: Mature, bone-forming cells.

peristalsis: The wavelike contractions of smooth muscle in the digestive system.

sprain: An injury caused by stretched ligaments.

strain: An injury caused by damage to muscles or tendons around a joint.

tendon: The connective tissue that attaches muscles to bones, cartilage, and other connective tissue.

vertebrae: The bones that make up the spinal column.

FOR FURTHER READING

Elizabeth Fong, *Body Structures and Functions*. St. Louis, MO: Times Mirror/Mosby, 1987. This book provides simple and thorough descriptions of various diseases of the human body.

David E. Larson, *Mayo Clinic Family Health Book*. New York: William Morrow, 1996. This book describes in simple terms the many diseases that can affect the human body.

Mary Lou Mulvihill, *Human Diseases*. Norwalk, CT: Appleton and Lange, 1995. This book provides a good description of the most common diseases of the human body.

World Book Medical Encyclopedia. Chicago: World Book, 1995. This book provides a vast amount of information on the physiology of the human body systems.

WORKS CONSULTED

Books

Robert Berkow, *The Merck Manual of Medical Information*. New York: Pocket Books, 1997. This book provides a detailed explanation of all organs and gives information on the causes, symptoms, diagnosis, and treatment of many diseases.

Charlotte Dienhart, *Basic Human Anatomy and Physiology*. Philadelphia: W.B. Saunders, 1979. This textbook covers the structure and function of all organ systems in the human body. It also provides information on symptoms and treatments of various diseases.

Arthur C. Guyton, *The Textbook of Medical Physiology*. Philadelphia: W.B. Saunders, 1991. This textbook relates anatomy and physiology to medical conditions.

John Hole Jr., *Essentials of Human Anatomy and Physiology*. Dubuque, IA: Wm. C. Brown, 1992. This textbook of anatomy and physiology provides detailed explanations of the structure and function of all human body systems.

Elaine Marieb, *Human Anatomy and Physiology*. Redwood City, CA: Benjamin/Cummings, 1995. This book offers a detailed explanation of all human body structures and organs.

Websites

About (www.about.com). This easy-to-use website offers information on all topics, including health and medicine.

About Children's Health (www.aboutchildrenshealth.com). This website contains good information about all types of body systems.

American Academy of Family Physicians (www.aafp.org). This website describes a variety of diseases and their treatments.

American Academy of Orthopaedic Surgeons (www.aaos.org). This website provides descriptions of orthopedic diseases and treatments.

BBC Health (www.bbc.co.uk). This is a good resource for health information.

CDC (www.cdc.gov). This website provides information from the national Centers for Disease Control and Prevention on any topic in health.

Children's Health (www.medem.com). Information on all types of children's health issues is supplied by Medem, Inc.

Clinical Implications (www.nobel.se). This website contains drawings and photographs along with information on all medical topics.

Cornell Medical College (www.edcenter.med.cornell.edu). The medical college of Cornell provides a wide range of information on body systems.

Countdown for Kids Magazine (www.jdf.org/kids/cfk). Students can research topics that interest them, including health and medicine.

11th Hour (www.blackwellscience.com). This is a valuable resource for any type of information in science.

Fact Monster, Learning Net Work (www.factmonstser.com). This website provides information in all topics; suitable for any student. It also provides a good science encyclopedia.

JAMA HIVAIDS Resource Center (www.ama-assn.org). The *Journal of the American Medical Association*, published by the American Medical Association, is a great resource for any topic in medicine.

The Merck Manual Website (www.merck.com). This website gives a detailed explanation of body systems and diseases.

MSN Search (www.search.msn.com). This website provides a science library suitable for most students.

Top Condition (http://topcondition.com). This website contains an extensive collection of articles on all aspects of the musculoskeletal system.

Yucky Kids (www.nj.com/yucky). This website provides easy-to-read articles on a variety of science topics.

Internet Sources

ABC News.com, "High Hopes for Hips," 2002. http://abcnews.go.com.

About, "What Are Common Knee Problems?" 2002. http://sports medicine.about.com.

Advanced Medical Technology Association, "Ultrasound Device for Healing Bone Fractures," 2002. www.himanet.com.

American Academy of Orthopaedic Surgeons, "Fractures," 2002. http://orthoinfo.aaos.org/all.cfm.

Elixir Industry, "Start Investing in Your Bones Today," 2002. www.elixir industry.com.

Geocities, "Are You Double Jointed?" 2002. www.geocities.com.

How Stuff Works, "How Exoskeletons Work," 2002. www.howstuff works.com.

Personal Trainer, "The Knee," 2002. www.topcondition.com.

Science for Seniors, "Novel Form of Vitamin D Shown to Grow Bone," 2002. www.scienceforseniors.org.

Science News Online, "Marrow Transplant Fights Bone Disease," 2002. www.sciencenews.org.

Space Medicine and Life Sciences Research Center, "Musculoskeletal Research," 2002. www.msm.edu.

United States Bone and Joint Decade News, "Why Is the Bone and Joint Decade Important?" 2002. www.usbjd.org.U.S. Food and Drug Administration, "Help for People with Paget's Disease," 2002. www.fda.gov.

INDEX

PICTURE CREDITS

ABOUT THE AUTHORS

Both Pam Walker and Elaine Wood have degrees in biology and education from colleges in Georgia. They have taught science in grades seven through twelve since the mid–1980s.

Ms. Walker and Ms. Wood are coauthors of more than a dozen science teacher resource activity books and two science textbooks.